THE COMPLETE GUIDE TO ANTI-AGING NUTRIENTS

SHELDON SAUL HENDLER
M.D., PH.D.

Simon and Schuster   New York

Published by Simon and Schuster
A Division of Simon & Schuster, Inc.
Simon & Schuster Building
Rockefeller Center
1230 Avenue of the Americas
New York, New York 10020

SIMON AND SCHUSTER and colophon are registered trademarks
of Simon & Schuster, Inc.

Designed by J. Nichols & R. Ottiger/Levavi & Levavi

Manufactured in the United States of America

Library of Congress Cataloging in Publication Data

Hendler, Sheldon Saul.
    The Complete Guide to Anti-Aging Nutrients.

    Includes index.
    1. Nutrition. 2. Health. 3. Dietary supplements.
4. Longevity—Nutritional aspects. I. Title.
RA784.H45 1984   613.2   84-23469
ISBN: 0-671-50615-3

ACKNOWLEDGMENTS

I must first thank my wife, Joyce, who shared many sleepless nights with me during the writing of this book.

I am indebted to my colleagues and friends at Mercy Hospital and Medical Center in San Diego for their encouragement and support. With special thanks to Drs. Stewart Frank, Jack Geller, Stanley Amundson, and Richard Kornberg and Mr. John Reilly.

My gratitude to Drs. Lissy Jarvik, Yasuo Hotta, Adrian Barbul, Gordon Gill, Peter Hornsby, and A. M. Michelson for sharing with me the results of their most interesting studies, and to Mark McCarty and Dr. Alex Mercandetti for inspiring conversations.

Finally, special thanks and affection to my agent, D.M.R. of Proteus Inc., who taught me how to write a book.

To the memory of:

Dr. Sol Spiegelman, father of molecular biology, good friend and constant source of inspiration, and my parents, Rose and Alexander Hendler. All should have lived much longer than they did.

CONTENTS

SEPARATING
FACT
FROM
FICTION

Nutritional
"True Believers"
vs. "Academic
Conservatives"

For years, friends and colleagues familiar with my background as a biochemical researcher and, more recently, as a medical doctor with a strong interest in human metabolism, diet and nutrition have asked me where they could find objective, reliable, scientific information on vitamins, minerals and other food supplements. Among their questions were these: Which supplements, if any, are worth taking? Is there evidence suggesting that these supplements do any good? How sound is the evidence? What is the source of it? Which substances appear to be safe—and in what doses? Which are the best forms in which to take the various supplements? Which are the best combinations? What results can be expected? Who should take supplements—and when? Should everyone take the same thing or should different people of different ages and in different life situations follow different regimens? Can the claims of the supplement manufacturers and those contained in health-food-store handouts, popular books and so on be believed?

I felt compelled to examine carefully the information that was available to the general public and to the typical physician. I was distressed and, quite frankly, depressed by what I found. On the one hand, I encountered the old-line nutritional "academic conservatives" who doggedly go on insisting that the "balanced American diet" will provide the right amounts of fat, carbohydrates and protein as well as all of the vitamins, minerals and other micronutrients anyone could possibly need. The data attesting to the awful toll the "balanced American diet" has taken on us are becoming overwhelming. As a nation we are overfed and often seriously undernourished. Dietary/nutritional imbalances and deficiencies contribute significantly to the premature deaths of millions of Americans annually. Moreover, our changing world has placed new demands on our bodies, exposing them to environmental stresses and insults that were not previously so prevalent, stresses and insults that deplete our tissues of protective micronutrients as never before.

And, on the other hand, I encountered what I will call the nutritional "true believers," those who tout or regard every new supplement that comes along as some sort of miracle substance or panacea. The true-believer category, unfortunately, almost certainly includes a good many who may not believe so much in the efficacy of the products they sell as they do in the ability of those products, if hyped loud enough and long enough, to generate big profits. The supplement supermarket is now ringing up more than $3 billion in revenues annually. It is big business. And every sort of opportunist has moved in for part of the kill.

Poorly researched, self-serving books, magazines, brochures and advertising handouts abound—all aimed at convincing the consumer that he or she will be happier, healthier, sexier, slimmer, more energetic, smarter and longer-lived if only he or she will buy this particular product or formula. Many of the authors of these enthusiastic books and articles, despite claims to the contrary, have suspect or insufficient credentials for the tasks they have assigned themselves. Many of the major vitamin and mineral companies do not have even a single reputable research scientist on their staffs, although, interestingly, many of the major pharmaceutical companies are now researching and producing vitamin and mineral supplements in recognition of the fact that literally tens of millions of Americans in a variety of categories are in need of micronutrient supplementation.

In the middle—between the true believers and the academic conservatives—I found very little. So I set out to research and write a book that would, without any axe to grind, without any products to sell or any vested interests to protect, systematically and objectively analyze the scientific data available for each of the micronutrients and other substances for which *anti-aging* claims have been made.

I stress "anti-aging" because that term encompasses most of the important claims. Most of the disease processes, as well as the decline in sexual performance, energy and so on, are ultimately seen to be part and parcel of the overall aging phenomenon that everyone—me included—wants to slow down. The book that seemed to me to be so badly needed—and the one that I have tried to write—is a genuine consumer's guide to these so-called anti-aging nutrients and other food supplements.

My approach has been as objective and pragmatic as I could make it. I have sought always to be guided by the best available data. If something seems to work, I don't hesitate to say so; and if something clearly doesn't work or is unsafe, I am not reluctant to reveal that either. In many cases, I am compelled to say that we still don't know or we will have to wait for more research before a particular substance can be declared safe or efficacious. Though better information is emerging all the time and though we now have a body of data that can be quite useful if properly interpreted and utilized, it is wise to remember that our knowledge concerning the effects micronutrients can have on human health remains incomplete.

Good News Without Exaggeration

The literature that characterizes the true-believer school of nutrition is replete with bad science, selective use of the data, half-baked hypotheses, unreliable "anecdotal" evidence, mistaken conclusions, gross misunderstandings of basic biochemistry and human metabolism, misinterpretation and, especially, gross exaggeration. This exaggeration is a product of a combination of things, principally ignorance, wishful thinking and often greed. It is the ignorance that is particularly worrisome, for it is an ignorance that shortchanges the consumer *twice*, once by claiming things that simply aren't true or can't be substantiated and then once again by completely missing benefits that might legitimately be claimed.

Time and again, as you will see, I find nutrients and supplements being touted for all the wrong reasons—entirely without scientific support—while some genuine "indications" for these same substances, indications buttressed by sound research data, go entirely overlooked. This is highly significant, not only in terms of respecting the facts, but in terms also of practical application of these substances. The reason *why* you take a supplement has, logically, a great deal to do with *who* should take it, *when* it should be taken, *how much* should be taken, what it should be taken *with*, and so on. It is vitally important, therefore, to know, first and foremost, whether the claimed indication or reason for using any given nutrient is valid.

This book sharply focuses on those "indications" and "reasons." It highlights the good news—but always and only the good news that can be supported by reliable scientific findings. And this book does not shrink from calling attention to some bad news, that is, to things that don't work or are unsafe. Even this, however, is really good news for the discriminating consumer. Knowing what *won't* help you or might even harm you is just as useful as knowing what will help.

The wonderful thing about this area of research is that, if you know how to find it, there is so much that is exciting and promising that even the most ardent enthusiast need not resort to exaggeration in order to deliver plenty of good news. The *facts* are exciting enough in their own right. Let's insist on those facts. That's the only way that the excesses and oversights of the true believers can be vanquished and the skepticism of the academic conservatives, who continue to control so much of the research, can be overcome.

The good news that this book imparts can be summarized as follows: There are no quick fixes or "magic bullets" or miracle combinations of nutrients that will enable you to underexercise and overindulge and still remain youthful into advanced age.

There is no formula that will let you extend your life-span beyond that maximum which Mother Nature has genetically foreordained. Anyone who claims otherwise is selling snake oil, no matter what he labels it.

However, there *is* plenty you can do to reach your maximum life-span, that is, to live out more of your genetic potential, and, moreover, to do so in reasonably good health almost until the end. Most of us don't make it beyond our early seventies, and even then the last decades of our lives are often plagued by innumerable complaints related to physical degeneration. Before we begin worrying about breaking the maximum life-span barrier and living to be 140 or 1,040, shouldn't we try to figure out how to make it to 110 (which, for most of us, is probably the genetic limit) in good health and free of most of those typical "old-age" complaints?

We stand a good chance of being able to do just that. We can't put off death indefinitely, but we *can* compress morbidity. What this means is that we can extend average life-span and shorten the period in which we suffer the infirmities ("morbidities") of old age to a brief period just before we die. We have among us a significant number of individuals who live into their eighties and nineties and even beyond with remarkable vigor and with relatively youthful appearance, individuals whose cardiovascular systems and mental faculties are, by objective standards and testing, the equal of those of healthy people in their thirties and forties. Why can't we *all* be like that or even better, proceeding to 100 or even to 110 in many cases with strength, energy, optimism?

The answer is that we can, using our current knowledge of nutrition and especially micronutrition. Exercise and stress management are important factors that can help compress morbidity. Diet and nutrition are perhaps even more important factors. And it is those nutritional factors that this book focuses upon in particular, especially vitamins, minerals and other food supplements. These are not magic bullets, but they are potent weapons, when used properly, in the battle against premature aging.

What's in This Book?

Part One of this book tells you what aging *is* and, equally important, what it *isn't*. The good news here is that much of what we have come to believe to be an inevitable part of aging is actually *preventable*—if we take care of ourselves and especially if we are careful about diet and nutrition. The most persuasive theories of aging are reviewed with the objective of gaining insight into ways we might combat aging.

Part One then proceeds to examine the effects of diet and nutrition on aging. The impact of both macronutrition and micronutrition is analyzed. Guidelines based on the best available current scientific data are provided for fats, carbohydrates and protein, as well as such other macronutrient components as fiber, salt, added sugar, etc. Changes in diet that are the most likely to enhance our health, primarily through the prevention or amelioration of the major degenerative diseases, including cancer and cardiovascular disease, are summarized.

Part Two is devoted to detailed analyses of the micronutrients and other food supplements. Nearly every substance for which some significant anti-aging claim has been made is analyzed in Part Two. Here you will find most of the vitamins and minerals, the amino acids, nucleic acids, fats and lipids, various pharmaceuticals and chemicals, and a wide variety of popular food supplements, as well as many newly emerging supplements. The claims for each substance, both pro and con, are reviewed and then examined against the best available scientific evidence from around the world. Then, based on those data, I make my recommendations. In the course of preparing these analyses, I have read literally thousands of research papers.

Part Three of the book proposes a number of micronutrient regimens for individuals in different life situations, including "basic" preventive regimens for generally healthy men and women, special regimens for smokers, alcohol drinkers, women on the Pill, pregnant women, postmenopausal women, surgical patients, people on weight-loss diets, athletes, etc. Part Three also provides information on the relative merits and demerits of "one-a-day," "insurance," "stress" and other special formulas, and answers questions related to the labeling of products, the best forms in which to buy them, the "synthetic" versus "natural" controversy and so on.

Read in good health *and* long life.

PART ONE

NUTRITION AND AGING

The Promising New Findings

one

HOW LONG CAN WE LIVE?

"Die young/Stay pretty."

What is aging? I asked a group of young schoolchildren this question, and here are some of the often illuminating answers I got: "Growing up." "Getting old." "Wrinkles." "Getting sick and having to go to the hospital all the time." "Being too tired to tell stories." "Dyeing your hair." "Playing golf a lot." "Forgetting things." "Retiring." "False teeth." "Having a bad temper." "Trouble hearing." "Dying." And, from one precocious youngster: "Fermentation."

I then asked: Is there anything we can do to stop or slow down aging? Some of the answers: "Put on lots of makeup." "Get a face-lift." (Enthusiastically seconded by several of the other children.) "Go to the doctor." "Dye your hair." "Jog like my father does." "Wear nice clothes." "Take pills." "Take vitamins." "Get lots of rest so you don't wear out so fast." "Brush after

every meal." "Eat good foods." And from the precocious one:
"Don't grow up."

That last answer reminded me of a line from a song that was
popular among teenagers a while back: "Die young/stay pretty,"
which was perhaps inspired by a much earlier line from a Hum-
phrey Bogart movie—"Live fast, die young and have a good
lookin' corpse."

Most of these answers were delivered amid bursts of nervous
giggles—early eruptions of the sort of gallows humor with which
most of us, alas, still approach the—pun intended—grave issue
of aging. Our view of this universal phenomenon continues, for
the most part, pessimistic, indeed, fatalistic. Almost all of us
believe that aging is inevitable and, though we are often reluctant to say so out loud, we further believe, on the basis of personal experience and/or observation, that the process is almost
always unpleasant, that it is often painful and immobilizing, and
that it is usually—horror of horrors—*unsightly*.

It is not terribly difficult to maintain these beliefs, for we are
continually bombarded with grim statistics attesting to our awful
mortality. Arthritis, heart disease, cancer and the other degenerative diseases and disorders associated with the aging process
are continually in the news. One in three adult male Americans
dies of heart disease; 1,000 people in the U.S. alone die of cancer
each day; nursing homes and retirement centers are popping up
all around us; Medicare is in constant funding trouble; aging
costs the economy billions of dollars annually, etc. etc.

And, of course, as the ultimate reminder of our mortality, our
friends and relatives continue to die.

What is aging anyway, and does it really have to be so awful?
These are some of the questions this chapter will attempt to
answer.

It is widely accepted among scientists that our maximum life-
span—the full genetic *potential* beyond which we cannot go
without engineering a fundamental change in our genetic
makeup—is about 110 years. Some argue—but without scientific evidence—that we might actually have the capacity to live
to be 130 or 140. We've all heard stories of isolated individuals
or particularly hardy groups in remote areas of the world who
are supposed to have attained these hoary ages, but these
claims, when carefully scrutinized, have, unfortunately, *always*
proved false. Hunzas, living in the villages of the Russian Cau-
casus, for example, have claimed to be 130 to 160, but a sober

investigation by Zhores Medvedev, a Soviet gerontologist, revealed fake Methuselahs who were actually in their seventies and eighties, though many of them, after particularly arduous lives, *looked* as if they could be 140! (See *The Gerontologist*, 14:381, 1974.)

Few of us will make it to age 100; not many of us will even make it to ninety. Improved standards of living (including better nutrition and sanitary conditions) have enabled more of us to live longer—extending *average* life-span from forty-seven years to seventy-three years in this century—but have done absolutely nothing to extend *maximum* life-span. It should be noted, however, that if a man makes it to age seventy, he can, on average, expect to live another eleven years; women who attain that age can, on average, expect to live another fourteen years. Both men and women who make it to age eighty can expect, on average, to live another six years. As indicated above, and as will be explored in more detail later, there is little chance that we will be able to extend *maximum* life-span any time soon. We can, however, add years of good health to our lives—within the confines of maximum life-span. With increased knowledge, of the sort that is rapidly accumulating and is the focus of much of this book, many of us can achieve more of our full-life potentials.

And with this same increased knowledge we can make those added years *good* years, years relatively free of the degenerative processes that presently plague our senior population. There is no sense in trying to extend maximum life-span until we have made the most of what is already allotted us, until we can live out a significant number of those 110 years in reasonably good health, in happiness, and in possession of both mental and physical vitality. The idea, as explained in the Introduction to this book, must be to *compress morbidity* to that period immediately preceding death. It is presently mostly a waste of time to dream about living to be 140, let alone 1,040. But it is definitely *not* nonsense to aim to live to be 90, 100 or even 110 and to aim, moreover, to do so in generally good health right up until near the end.

Compression of morbidity—retarding the worst manifestations of aging for as long as possible—is what this book ultimately addresses. Even the schoolchildren I "polled" have begun to understand that this is our best hope. Their answers to my questions about slowing down aging were not entirely negative. They—and the public at large—have begun to perceive that our life-styles—and especially our eating and exercising habits—can, if modified, have definite, *positive* effects on the degenerative disorders that do so much to make us feel and look bad as we grow older.

But if we are really to understand why this is so, we must first understand what aging involves, not just its symptoms ("wrinkles," "forgetting things," etc.), but also its underlying mechanisms. Many of the things that we typically believe are inevitable parts of aging turn out, often, to be retardable or actually *avoidable*.

What Happens to Our Bodies When We Age? (First, Some Good News)

Aging is a gradual process that, when large populations are studied, follows *some* predictable paths. Do not conclude from this, however, that what happens in general must always happen in particular—to *every* individual at each chronological age. There have been only a very few good long-term studies of the aging process. One of the best of these is the Baltimore Longitudinal Study of Aging sponsored by the federal government's National Institute on Aging at its Gerontology Center. It started in 1958 and has been monitoring the aging process—via regularly conducted physical and psychological tests—in more than 1,500 individuals. One of its most important findings has related to the sometimes dramatic *variability* of aging in different people. Other researchers have documented this variability, as well, reporting, for example, that some seventy- and eighty-year-olds have healthier—i.e., *younger*—cardiovascular systems than some forty- or even thirty-year-olds.

In fact, the Baltimore Study has revealed that the older person's heart—if disease-free—can pump just about as well as the young adult's. This is a highly significant finding for it indicates that a failing heart is not an inevitable and intrinsic part of getting older. Keep constantly in mind the fact that so much of what we attribute to aging is actually the product of accumulated insults we heap on ourselves, in the form, for example, of bad nutrition, smoking, drinking to excess, exercising too little, and so on. In other words, much of what we call aging actually has to do with *how* we live more than with *how long* we live.

There's more good news of the same sort. You've probably heard since school days that your brain cells are dying at an alarming rate starting at an early age. Ten thousand or more of these cells, it is often claimed, bite the dust every day—until we are finally reduced to fumbling forgetfulness or even outright senile dementia. This brain-shriveling effect, we are further warned, is relentless and irreversible. This nonsense is still being spouted even by some doctors and reported upon in popular science magazines.

Recent research shows that while changes certainly do take place in the brain as we age, they are by no means so severe or intractable as the enduring pessimists would have us believe. A 10 percent decrease in brain volume has been observed, most of it occurring after age sixty, but it has never really been proved that this is accounted for by brain-cell loss. There is, if anything, more evidence that this decrease in volume is due to diminished extracellular spaces. Some of the brain cells unquestionably undergo degeneration, though even many of these, far from "giving up" or dying, often seem to retain significant function.

The Baltimore Study has shown that memory loss is very mild through the middle years of healthy individuals and that the healthy elderly are as good at remembering such things as seven-digit telephone numbers as are the young. Some extremely healthy old people (including some in their nineties, according to research findings of the National Institute of Mental Health) have oxygen consumption in, and blood flow through, the brain equal to that of healthy people *fifty* years younger. These oldsters usually demonstrate memories and reasoning powers that are also the equal of much younger, healthy individuals. Even looking at the general population, rather than at the extremely healthy, the Baltimore Study finds that reasoning ability does not diminish significantly until quite late in life.

Equally encouraging is the growing conviction among researchers that the brain possesses remarkable "plasticity," that it can grow as well as regress, even as we age, and that, in fact, it can reverse direction in response to a number of environmental and psychological factors. After reviewing some 140 studies on the relationships of aging and the extent to which various physical and mental properties are used, Dr. Walter Bortz of the Palo Alto (California) Medical Clinic concluded that people who use their memories and other mental faculties the most lose them the least. This conclusion is consistent with the results of animal studies in which rats placed in "enriched" environments with lots of stimulation lived significantly longer than normal and were found to have cerebral cortexes and dendritic (brain cell) growth as extensive as much younger animals.

Recently, Dr. Lissy Jarvik, Chief of Psycho-geriatrics at the Brentwood Veterans Administration Medical Center in Los Angeles, similarly reported (personal communication, 1984) that mental exercise may be as important to the maintenance of the brain as physical exercise is to the maintenance of the body. Those aging men and women who kept most mentally active were the ones, in Dr. Jarvik's long-term study, who were most likely to retain their thinking/cognitive abilities. The mental activity required, she told the LA Times/Washington Post News Service, "could be reading the newspaper, listening to the news, reading books or magazines, playing cards or playing shuffleboard. It doesn't have to be something esoteric; it could be anything that keeps a person from getting into a total rut." The idea is to find activities that are personally involving or challenging.

And here's still more good news: The Baltimore Study has found that many, in fact *most*, older men who are in good health continue to make the hormones that are essential for male sexual functioning. And they make them in quantities generally *equal* to those produced by younger men. Others have noted a "use it or lose it" component in sexual functioning. Those who use it most use it longer and later in life.

You will notice that in the foregoing discussion there is an emphasis on "good health" as a prerequisite for retaining into old age many of the body's most vital functions. Getting and keeping "good health" embraces a number of factors over which we, individually, exert a good deal of control. Diet and exercise are two of the most important of these factors. The point is, if we take care of ourselves, many of the processes that we have falsely come to believe are inevitable results of getting older can be slowed down or even largely avoided. This book, in subsequent chapters, focuses, especially, on the role various dietary nutrients and other food supplements can play in helping us to stay in good health and thus to compress morbidity.

Then Some Bad News
(but not all that bad)

Some of you may be thinking, No matter how well we live, we're still going to die eventually. True. One must acknowledge the inconstancy of the flesh. No matter how conscientiously we seek to preserve it, it will eventually give out on us. Still, the research cited above proves it doesn't have to give out as quickly as most believe; it can remain relatively strong into advanced age. The widely observed, generalized declines in various systems of the body that are summarized below do not show what *must* happen; instead they show what *often* happens in significant part because of our unhealthy life-styles (smoking, drinking, lack of exercise, poor nutrition and so on).

Let's look at the major parts of the body and review some of the changes that are frequently observed with aging.

HEART AND LUNGS—Pumping efficiency of the heart especially during exercise typically diminishes as we age; vital capacity of the lungs is impaired and diffusion of oxygen is reduced. Blood flow is decreased, and the capacity for physical work is diminished. Increasing stiffness of the arteries is observed, and there is an increase, generally, in systolic blood pressure. Given the fact, however, that healthy hearts and lungs have been found in men even older than one hundred years places in doubt many of those grim figures that confidently project sizable declines in function between certain ages. Declines of those types and magnitude need *not* apply to many of those who keep themselves healthy through diet, exercise, etc.

BRAIN AND NERVOUS SYSTEM—There is a thickening of the meninges, the membranes that envelop the brain and spinal cord; brain volume diminishes by about 10 percent between ages thirty and seventy. Deficits in short-term memory and learning ability, depression, withdrawal, rigidity of outlook and dementia are increasingly observed, especially after age sixty. Velocity of nerve signal transmission diminishes, as does sensory awareness. Production of brain neurotransmitters decreases with age. Reflexes slow. Again, however, there is evidence that many of these age-related phenomena can be retarded through improved nutrition, mental exercise and so on.

HORMONES/METABOLISM—Metabolic rate slows with age; composition of the body typically changes, with fat usually increasing. Thyroid function declines. Glucose tolerance diminishes with age, and the incidence of both diabetes and obesity increases. Thymic hormones, involved in immune function, begin to decline soon after puberty. Estrogen levels fall sharply in women, producing menopause, usually in the early fifties; lack of estrogen predisposes women to increased rate of bone loss (osteoporosis). Again, exercise and diet can slow down/reduce many of the hormonal/metabolic age-related changes.

MUSCLE—Muscular strength typically peaks in the mid-twenties; decline in muscular strength is often evident in the mid-forties. By the mid-sixties, muscular strength is frequently half of what it was in the mid-twenties. Loss of coordination accompanies loss of muscular strength. This form of debilitation, however, can be largely forestalled well into later life through exercise. There are sixty-year-olds who have greater muscular strength and better coordination than do some twenty- and thirty-year-olds. "Use it or lose it" definitely applies here.

SKELETON—Vertebral disks often begin deteriorating in the thirties, and some loss of height may be noted already in this decade. Thinning of bone, loss of joint elasticity, degeneration of cartilage and ligaments all increase with age, as does the incidence of osteophytosis (formation of bony spurs), arthritis, osteoporosis, and other bone and joint diseases. By age sixty, loss of up to an inch in height is commonly noted due to degeneration of bones and joints. Vulnerability to fractures increases with age. That's the grim picture that is commonly presented in texts on aging. But, in fact, many of these degenerative changes can be forestalled and even eliminated with good nutrition and regular exercise.

GASTROINTESTINAL SYSTEM—Slow wasting of the intestinal glands contributes to increasing difficulties with digestion and absorption. The incidence of peptic ulcers, constipation, diverticulosis, malnutrition increases with age. Diseases of the teeth, gums and jaw also typically increase. (You will find, in subsequent chapters, nutritional approaches to slowing down some of these processes.)

GENITOURINARY SYSTEM—The nephrons, the functional units of the kidneys, are reduced in number as we age. So is blood flow into and out of the kidneys, though by how much remains uncertain. The reduction may not be nearly so great as was once believed if generally good health is maintained.

As some of the above suggests, the major diseases associated with the aging processes are:

1. CANCERS—Our chances of getting one form of cancer or another double every eight years that we continue to live beyond the age of forty-five. Problems of immunity, breakdown in cellular repair mechanisms, increased exposure to cancer-causing agents, the accumulated effects of poor nutrition and other factors all combine to make cancer an age-related phenomenon, though *not* an inevitable one.

2. CARDIOVASCULAR DISEASE—The incidences of heart attacks, strokes, coronary-artery disease, etc. all increase steadily with the passage of years. Multiple factors contribute: dietary overindulgence, nutritional deficiencies, lack of exercise, smoking, excessive drinking, high blood pressure, diabetes.

3. ARTHRITIS—The relationship of bone and joint disorders to aging has to do with accumulated wear and tear over time and also with factors related to immune response and, some evidence suggests, diet and nutrition.

4. DIABETES—The incidence of adult diabetes increases significantly after age thirty and goes on increasing thereafter; there is a doubling every ten years in one's chances of getting this disease after age thirty. Hormonal, metabolic, immune and dietary factors all play roles in this age-related risk.

5. SENILE DEMENTIA—Generally associated with very advanced age, various forms of dementia are now known to afflict, to varying degrees, large numbers of individuals, some as young as their forties. Again, nutritional deficiencies may play a cumulative role in these disorders, along with age-related disturbances in and shortages of the brain's neurotransmitters, which are also affected by diet. Degeneration of brain cells is another factor, though, as previously noted, brain cells do not die off at

the prodigious rate once believed. And brain "exercises," also discussed previously, can help keep the mind alert.

6. IMMUNE-RELATED DISORDERS AND DISEASES—Susceptibility to infections and autoimmune diseases, as well as to cancer, increases with age. Various cells of the immune system are dependent for growth, development and optimal functioning upon certain hormones, the production of which generally declines with age.

It is very difficult to establish what parts/functions of the body will age—and at what precise stages—*independent* of anything we might do to try to "optimize" nutrition, exercise, etc. It *is* clear, however, that many of the degenerative processes and diseases that were believed to be inevitable, intrinsic manifestations of aging *can* be forestalled or avoided and that it *is* possible to live into advanced age relatively free of these disorders.

Theories of Aging

So far we have mostly been considering the *effects* of aging. We know quite a bit about some of those but far less about *why* we age. There has been no dearth of *theories* to try to explain aging nor any lack of effort to try to unify these theories in order to project a master-control mechanism or "clock" that governs all the myriad manifestations of aging. So far, no one theory has persuaded the scientific community of its primacy; nor has anyone yet succeeded in locating "the clock of aging," let alone in setting back its dials (except within the context of what appears to be our genetically programmed "maximum life-span"). New findings are emerging all the time, however, and we do now possess information that makes it possible for us to begin slowing down aging in the sense that is most realistic at the present time—via the compression of morbidity that we have been discussing.

For a long time it was believed that the mechanisms that govern the rate of aging were located outside the cells. The prevailing theory today, however, is that the clock of aging is inside the cells themselves. Gerontologist Leonard Hayflick has demonstrated—and many others have confirmed—that normal human cells have finite lifetimes of about fifty population doublings when grown in laboratory cultures. This finitude has come to be known throughout the world as "the Hayflick Limit." If you freeze cells after thirty doublings, then thaw them out and put them back in culture, they will proceed to divide again—doubling about twenty more times. The precision of the Hayflick Limit is quite impressive. If you put the cells of older people in culture you'll find, for example, that they have far fewer doublings left in them than do the cells of younger people. The same applies to the cells of those afflicted with diseases or conditions (such as Mongolism) that program them for premature deaths. More and more correlations are being made between the number of cell doublings in culture and maximum life-spans in a great many animals. (See *Scientific American* 242:58, 1980.)

Dr. Hayflick's work has helped open the way for an intensive search for the clock of aging—within the cells themselves. Researchers are now literally taking cells apart and then reassembling them in an effort to locate the clock. They have put young nuclei—containing all the genetic information in the cell—into old cells, after having first removed the nuclei of those old cells; and then, by growing these reassembled cells in culture, they have proved that the clock is located somewhere in the nucleus and not in the cytoplasm (outer portion of the cell). Now they are introducing individual chromosome pairs from old cells into the nuclei of young cells. If the cells thus altered die sooner than expected, they will know that they have located the chromosome or chromosomes upon which the clock is situated. Soon the search will focus on the still smaller genes that constitute the clock itself.

What all of this tells us is that aging appears to be "programmed," that it is a phenomenon encoded within our genes. Events may occur at higher biological hierarchies, within various of the organs, for example, but these too, according to the program theory, are governed by the genes. Our immune and endocrine (hormone) systems exert influences as we grow older that bring about various degenerative changes in our bodies. Some focus on these events and believe that they are themselves the mechanisms of aging. The best evidence, however, suggests that these hormonal and immunological events are merely "pacemakers," albeit important pacemakers, of aging, again governed by the instructions wound up in the genes of each cell. We may be able to live out more of our maximum life-span by manipulating some of these pacemakers, but if we want to actually *extend* maximum life-span, it appears that we will have to eventually learn how to reset the cellular genetic clock of aging.

The theories of aging that are most useful to us, from the standpoint of our being able to do something about them, are called "damage theories." Some people—most of us at one time or another—intuitively believe that we age simply because of "wear and tear," because "the works get gummed up" and we just "wear out." Damage accumulates over a lifetime and we finally lose the ability to adequately repair ourselves. These are the damage theories of aging, and though some people like to try to strictly separate them from the program theories, this really isn't possible. It all eventually comes back to the genes, which apparently fix the rate at which we can repair the damage inflicted upon us in the course of living. This doesn't mean, however, that the program doesn't give us some leeway, and possibly some significant leeway, some room in which we can actively take steps to avoid damage, reduce damage and help fix it when it does occur.

The damage theories hold that the genetic apparatus that directs every aspect of our development is bombarded by random insults that finally so mess up the program that it can no longer express enough of the life instructions to keep us going —and so we die. Does that mean, then, that if we could avoid damage altogether we'd live forever? The question is probably beside the point because the mere act of breathing—even pure air—inflicts some damage. So does normal, healthy metabolism. And nature seems to have programmed us in such a way that we can never quite repair the damage as fast as it occurs.

Aging, in some respects, appears to be a mere side effect of evolution. It is through damage and random "error" that new genetic combinations—mutations—arise. Sometimes these mutations have favorable effects, conferring advantages that make us more adaptable, more survivable in a changing environment, and are thus incorporated into the dynamic, ongoing genetic program. The longevity and survival of the species as a whole are thus paid for by the nonsurvival, the aging and the death of individuals within the whole. If we could repair all of the "errors" all of the time, evolution would come to a screeching halt.

I won't argue, however, that the next time one of your joints aches or you notice a new wrinkle that you should grin, bear it and congratulate yourself for having helped evolution do its job. For one thing, we are in the earliest emanations of a new epoch in which a living organism—man—perceives the ability of directing its own evolution, rather than leaving it to chance; and for another thing, I feel reasonably confident that Mother Nature and evolution will be able to tolerate our lack of passive cooperation.

There are a great many things that can inflict damage on our genetic programs. These include the air we breathe, the sun that our skin is exposed to, the food we eat, by-products of normal metabolism, free radicals (discussed below), pathogenic agents such as viruses and bacteria, enzyme imbalances, nutritional deficiencies, toxins and pollutants, radiation, etc. There are also many different places in the genetic machinery where the damage can strike. Life's essential instructions are encoded within the DNA—deoxyribonucleic acid—and are conveyed to the "messenger" RNA—ribonucleic acid—which, in turn, delivers these instructions to structures outside the cell nucleus called ribosomes. It is on the ribosomes that the instructions for protein synthesis, upon which all life depends, are carried out with the help of yet another form of RNA, called transfer RNA.

In the midst of all this complexity it is very easy to see how "errors" could arise and how, in sufficient numbers, they might prove debilitating or even deadly. Add to this "inside" vulnerability all the potential outside insults that can be heaped upon us, in the form of radiation, pollutants, bad diet, etc., and you may begin to marvel, as I do, that we operate as well as we do! If the instructions don't get lost or garbled somewhere along the way, the cell's energy-delivering furnaces—the mitochondria—might misfire or underfire; the ribosomes, even if sufficiently energized, may still break down in one way or another and produce defective proteins; or the cell's lysosomes, which enzymatically help break down the nutrients that feed the cells, may release too many enzymes at one time, disturbing or destroying the entire cell.

Damage theories may focus, from one authority to another, upon errors of DNA replication, errors of RNA transcription, ribosomal errors of protein synthesis, run-amok lysosomes and so on. The prevailing damage theories, however, fall into two categories discussed below.

THE CROSS-LINKING THEORY OF AGING (WHENCE COMES THE WORD "STIFF")—This is the "gummed-up" or "bound-and-gagged" theory of aging. Migrant molecules, which enter the body via foods, dietary liquids, air, especially polluted air, or which arise in the body as a result of normal metabolic processes, radiation and so on, are capable of attaching themselves to other molecules and linking them together. There is evidence that the body's ability to shake off these "cross-links" declines with age due to reduced enzyme-dissolving action and diminished free-radical scavenging (see below). Much of the basic stiffness and inelasticity of age is attributed to cross-linked molecules in the connective tissues. The more cross-linking there is, especially of the molecules close to the DNA helix, the more incapacitated we become, and incapacitation, according to this theory, yields to death when cross-linkage becomes so severe that the program can no longer adequately express itself. (For more on the important and influential cross-linking theory, see Bjorksten, *Chemistry*, 37:65, 1974, and Bjorksten, *Comprehensive Therapy*, 2:65, 1976.)

THE FREE-RADICAL THEORY OF AGING (LOOK OUT: ONE MIGHT LIKE YOU)—Free radicals are as wild as their name implies, but, actually, they don't like being "free," at least in the sense of remaining single or unattached. Free radicals are highly unstable, highly reactive molecules or fragments of molecules characterized by an unpaired free electron that is in a desperate tizzy to get hitched to almost anything it can grab. The gerontologist Alex Comfort has likened a free radical to "a convention delegate away from his wife: it's a highly reactive chemical agent that will combine with anything that's around." Science writer Albert Rosenfeld, in his book *Prolongevity* (Avon Books, New York, 1976), feels "combine" is too gentle a word and instead likens the free radical to a rapist, noting that "its union with another molecule . . . often amounts to an outright attack."

Free radicals are typically toxic oxygen molecules that severely damage most of the molecules they grab hold of (cell membranes and fat molecules are favorite targets). It is one of the fundamental ironies of life that oxygen both sustains us and kills us. We often forget how toxic oxygen is, though we need only look around us to be reminded of it. Most of the rust and decay that we encounter is due to oxidation. Much of the "rust and decay" of the human body is due to the same thing.

Yet we have an absolute requirement for oxygen. And the reason that we are able to live with it is that we segregate those oxygen reactions that would expose us to oxygen in its deadliest —singlet or hydroxyl free radical—form to specialized compartments of each cell we call the mitochondria (the respiratory, energy-producing centers of the cells). To help protect ourselves against the toxic forms of oxygen, such as superoxide, singlet oxygen, hydroxyl radicals, that spin off as a result of various metabolic processes, as well as those that enter the body in food or polluted air, or which form in the body as the result of radiation, viruses and so on, we arm ourselves with free-radical "scavengers."

Some of these scavengers are produced by the body in the form of enzymes, such as superoxide dismutase and glutathione peroxidase, names that will crop up from time to time in Part Two of this book. These enzymes break down and neutralize free radicals. So do a number of antioxidant substances, some of which are obtained in the diet—such as the mineral selenium and the vitamin ascorbic acid (vitamin C). If the free-radical scavengers are not present in sufficient quantity and at the right places at the right times, the free radicals can do considerable damage to the cells and to the genetic program itself. A certain amount of this kind of damage occurs almost all the time in each of us. Free radicals also help promote cross-linking, discussed above, and may help create destructive and sometimes malignant mutations. In polyunsaturated fats, free radicals help produce aldehydes and other substances that may produce cancer and other damage.

The free-radical theory of aging is probably the most useful theory we have at the present time—from the standpoint of finding practical means of delaying the effects of aging. Free radicals are something we can identify, measure and do battle with—especially through the sort of macro- and micronutritional regimens discussed in subsequent chapters of this book. For more on the free-radical theory of aging, see Harman, *American Journal of Clinical Nutrition*, 25:839, 1972, and Harman, *Proceedings of the National Academy of Sciences (U.S.—Biological Sciences)*, 78:7124, 1981.

Conclusion
(None of the Above . . .)

None of the above is the *one true* theory of aging. *All* have their merits and demerits. It seems highly likely that there *is* a genetic program that defines the outer limits of our longevity. The general assumption at the present time is that our maximum life-span is about 110 years of age—but no one *knows* this to be the case for sure; we believe it on the basis of the available, still inconclusive evidence.

Then, within the confines of maximum life-span, it appears certain that we have room to make our lives better by taking steps to prevent some of the diseases that are associated with but that are not, in fact, entirely synonymous with aging. It appears too, as will be evident later in this book, that we can take some important steps to protect against some of the specific damage attributed to cross-links and free radicals.

Will We Ever Live
Forever?

Most of this book is about things we can do right *now*, primarily through modification of diet and manipulation of micronutrient intake, to reduce or prevent some of the damage associated with aging. There are, however, some who want to do a whole lot more; there are some, in fact, who appear reluctant to settle for anything short of immortality—or at least a substantial extension of maximum life-span. Some of these ideas and efforts directed toward life everlasting deserve at least passing mention.

MAKING OLD CELLS YOUNG AGAIN—Some would-be immortalists have been excited by "cloning" experiments in which older cells that have already become highly specialized (as skin, bone, etc.) have been induced, in a sense, to become young again, behaving as if they were embryonic in origin and capable of giving rise to whole new organisms. In cloning experiments, the nuclei of body cells that have already differentiated into specific tissues have been transplanted into egg cells, the nuclei of which have been removed. In this environment, old nuclei have behaved as if they were young again. Instead of continuing as skin cells, liver cells or whatever it was they had differentiated into, they gave rise to whole new organisms, producing animals that were genetically identical to the animals from which the body-cell nuclei were taken. (See Gurdon, *The Control of Gene Expression in Animal Development*, Clarendon Press, Oxford, 1974.)

It should be understood that those working on cloning experiments have not been motivated by a desire to achieve immortality; they are interested in the mechanics of gene expression. But others have seen in this work evidence that the clock of aging *can* be reset to some extent. Others have speculated that organs might be cloned for transplantation whenever needed, extending life-span in that way.

REGENERATING MISSING OR DAMAGED PARTS—Some very exciting and fundamentally important work has been ongoing—and building—for many years in the realm of tissue regeneration stimulated by electromagnetic energy. In these experiments, as in some of the cloning experiments, it seems that ways are being discovered to give old cells a new lease on life, enabling them to perform functions that most of us would imagine were impossible. Cells seem to be capable of renewing themselves in some aspects when exposed to certain electromagnetic energies. Thus, researchers have achieved the regeneration of amputated limbs in some lower animals that don't normally have such regenerative capacities. Partial limb regeneration has even been achieved in some mammals (rats). (See Becker, *Nature*, 235:109, 1972; and Smith, *Annals of the New York Academy of Sciences*, 238:500, 1974.)

The life-spans of some single-celled organisms have been significantly extended in response to electromagnetic stimulation, and some recent research suggests that humans may benefit from certain electromagnetic manipulations as well, at least in terms of speeding healing of wounds and fractures. Some researchers believe electromagnetic stimulation may eventually be used to help damaged organs regenerate themselves—another approach to keeping us alive longer than might otherwise be expected.

LOOKING FOR THE "DEATH HORMONE"—The endocrine system, as discussed earlier, seems to constitute one of the major "pacemakers" of aging. There is ample evidence of age-related declines in the output and function of various hormones and hormone receptors in the body. Animal experiments are many in which the removal of a particular endocrine gland or the addition of a hormone or of a substance that modifies the activity of hormones seems to affect health, vigor and survival in a variety of ways. There have been reports (see, for example, Denckla, *Life Sciences*, 16:31, 1975) that aging is dramatically retarded in rats in which the pituitary glands have been removed. Some have speculated that there must be a "death hormone" produced by the pituitary, a substance that programs us for gradual decline and death. Removal of the pituitary is a drastic procedure—not recommended for humans or for any animal that will live outside a carefully maintained laboratory environment. Some are searching for an antidote to the hypothesized death hormone. This work is interesting but needs more follow-up. Most researchers continue to believe that while the pituitary may embrace one of the pacemakers of aging, the real clock remains out of easy reach within the DNA of each cell.

IMMUNOENGINEERING—Various aspects of the immune system seem to decline with age. Some of these deficits are related to decline in hormones that help regulate the body's defense mechanisms. Not only do we become more susceptible to infection and cancer as we grow older, but we also develop more "autoimmune" diseases in which some of the cells that had previously defended us now turn against us. In recent years, researchers have begun making progress in finding and describing the genetic components of immunity—that part of the total genetic program that orchestrates our defense systems. It is beginning to appear that the "command headquarters" of immunity may be concentrated in a manageable number of genes that may eventually—though not in the near future—be amenable to sophisticated immunoengineering. (For more details, see, for example, Smith and Walford, *Nature*, 270:727, 1977.)

LIVING LONGER BY EATING LESS—Clive McKay of Cornell University was the first to report, in the 1930s, that severe "caloric restriction" (underfeeding) can apparently extend the lifespans of various laboratory animals. Other researchers have since made similar reports, claiming that underfed animals (principally mice and rats) not only live longer than their better-fed brothers and sisters but that they develop fewer cancers and other age-related disorders. There is some indication that underfeeding slows the metabolic rate, delays sexual maturity (if started early), and influences other hormonal and immunological systems in ways that extend life-span. All of this work, however, remains highly speculative, particularly with respect to humans. And even the animal data have recently been called into question. It may very well be that underfed lab rats and mice are living no longer than their country cousins, who live in the wild state and also get far less to eat than the typical lab animal. Underfeeding may simply simulate conditions in the wild. No one knows how long wild mice/rats live if not prematurely killed by predators, adverse weather, etc. An increasing number of researchers are coming to the conclusion that "well-fed" lab animals are probably being *overfed*. And, as we know from human experience, being too well fed can lead to premature disease and death. Don't take seriously claims that a program of severe caloric restriction can help you live to be 120 or even 140; there's no scientific justification for these claims.

HIBERNATION AND THE DEEP FREEZE—There is some evidence that *cold-blooded* creatures can be persuaded to live longer than normal when they are kept at colder-than-normal temperatures. (See *American Journal of Clinical Pathology*, 74:247, 1980.) Some warm-blooded creatures of the human variety have decided that cooler temperatures might help them live longer too, though there is no scientific evidence of any substance to support this notion. As for efforts to prolong life via hibernation, those have yet to produce a truly useful yawn, though some animal experiments suggest that hibernative states may, eventually, be achieved in some species not ordinarily capable of hibernation. (See *Science*, 168:497, 1970, and *Cryobiology*, 15:113, 1978.) Some would-be immortalists have made arrangements to have their remains put "on ice" or "cryogenically suspended" at death, in hope that they can thus be preserved until a cure for whatever killed them comes along. I have a strong hunch these cool corpses-in-waiting will be waiting a very long time.

While some of the foregoing sounds fascinating—and some of it really is—don't start dreaming yet about the year 2100 (unless, perhaps, you're one or two years old *now*), let alone the year 3000. Immortality—or anything resembling it—is still the stuff of science fiction. We are, however, getting close to having our hands on the clock or clocks of aging. The danger isn't that we won't be able to find the clock but, rather, I submit, that we may find it *too soon*—before we're really prepared to understand it. Like a child puzzling over an intricate, delicate object, we may break something very important that we can't fix. We need to take time, among other things, to sort out the relative values of mortality and immortality. One thing is pretty certain: If we ever do achieve the ability to become immortal and decide to go for it, there probably will be no going back, and, like it or not, we'll then have all the time in the world to decide whether we did the right thing.

In the meantime, if you want to concentrate on things you can do right now—not to extend your maximum life-span but rather to live out more of it and in better health—read on.

two

MACRONUTRITION AND AGING (THE EFFECTS OF DIET AS A WHOLE)

Eat-Die (In Search of the Ideal Diet)

"Eat-Die." "Eat-Die." "Eat-Die." Imagine seeing those words in bold print repeated over and over. Your guess might be that you were reading an advertisement from an imaginative new horror film or looking at the front page of one of those supermarket tabloids. In fact, however, those words adorned the cover (Sept. 23, 1983) of the ordinarily unruffled journal *Science*, the official publication of the American Association for the Advancement of Science. A bit of scientific sensationalism from an unexpected quarter? Not at all. The article this eye-catching cover called quick attention to documented some of the emerging links between diet, aging and death.

The mere act of eating, even if we eat many of the right foods (and especially if we don't), increases the "opportunities" for aging. Normal metabolic processes, through which we break down foods in our bodies and derive energy from them, can produce a kind of toxic "exhaust" that takes the form of those free radicals discussed in the preceding chapter. When we eat the "wrong" foods, or too much of foods that might be good in moderation, when we are exposed to certain toxic additives and carcinogens in our foods, when foods aren't as fresh as they should be, when we eat a diet that fails to deliver adequate amounts of antioxidants and other protective and needed micronutrients, then the opportunities for aging increase even more.

When I talk about "macronutrition," I'm talking about the major components of diet—fat, protein, carbohydrates, all of which contain the vitamins and minerals and other "micronutrients" that are discussed in subsequent chapters of this book. In looking at diet as a whole, it is also wise to consider some other major players that influence aging: dietary fiber, salt, sugar, alcohol, smoking.

The typical American diet is often a series of disasters waiting to happen, It derives fully 40 percent of total calories from fats, and most of that fat is of the dangerous "saturated" variety that has been implicated in cardiovascular disease—the Number One killer in America—and in some forms of cancer. The typical American ingests 500 milligrams of cholesterol per day, two to five times what many heart experts say we should be getting. Those same experts advise that fat intake be limited to 20 percent of total calories and that no more than one-third of the fat be of the saturated variety.

Another basic problem with the standard American diet is its overreliance on refined carbohydrates, such as breads, cakes, etc. made of refined white flour and often liberally sweetened with sugar. Many nutrition experts now agree that carbohydrate intake should be increased overall—from the present 45 percent of total calories to about 65 percent of the total—but that emphasis should be placed on whole-grain and cereal products and on legumes (beans, peas, etc.). (See, for example, Connor and Connor, *Medical Clinics of North America,* 66:485, 1982). Not only will these *unrefined* complex carbohydrates add needed nutrients to the diet, they will also add bulk in the form of fiber. The typically overweight American often recoils at the thought of increasing carbohydrate intake, associating these macronutrients with weight gain. And, indeed, in refined form, carbohydrates do produce weight gain in many people. Unrefined carbohydrates, however, are likely to do just the opposite, adding bulk to the food and increasing the sensation of "satiety," of fullness, much more quickly and with fewer calories than can be achieved with fats, protein or refined carbohydrates. There is a growing consensus among nutritional experts that Americans need to increase fiber intake substantially—doubling it in many cases to 25 to 50 grams per day. Fruits, nuts and vegetables, along with grains and cereals, are good sources of fiber. (See discussion of fiber in Part Two for further details.) High-fiber diets not only contribute to weight loss and weight control but are also associated with a reduced incidence of diverticulosis and various forms of cancer. Some types of fiber, such as that found in oats, beans, apples and various other fruits, actually lower cholesterol levels in the blood.

About 15 percent of the calories in the American diet are derived from protein; most experts think it should stay at about that level. But there is growing agreement here too that the *source* of protein needs modification. Most of us, at present, get about 68 percent of our protein from animal sources. Research overall suggests that a healthier formula would be about 45 percent from vegetable sources and 55 percent from animal sources. This would simultaneously cut down on our intake of animal fats and increase our intake of fiber.

Alcohol must be considered too as part of the typical American diet. Two-thirds of the adult population indulges to some extent in alcohol. It's been estimated that among this population the typical drinker derives 8 to 22 percent of total calories from booze. These calories are largely empty of nutrients of the sort that protect against aging processes. And alcohol contains substances that produce carcinogens. (See cancer discussion below, which includes an evaluation of the impact of smoking on longevity, as well.)

The typical diet of the Western world has been associated with numerous degenerative diseases and aging processes. There is no question but that this diet promotes obesity, a condition that, when extreme, definitely predisposes us to heart disease, cancer, stroke, high blood pressure, diabetes and other disorders. It is also believed that the typical American diet adversely affects our immunity to disease and contributes, to some extent, to those autoimmune disorders such as rheumatoid arthritis. These links are strongly suggested by some research but have not yet been conclusively proved. To the extent that dietary factors—through the generation of free radicals, for example—undermine the genetic program that governs immunity, it is not difficult to conceive of ways in which the food we eat could impact on immunity, hormonal regulation and, in fact, every aspect of human life.

The best evidence that links diet to age-related diseases has to do with two of the major killers of our time—cancer and cardiovascular disease. These links are discussed below. They relate to ways in which diet can both contribute to and help prevent these diseases. What we learn from this evidence may have a great deal to do with the gradual construction of a new American diet. Some of what is discussed here is already having an impact in the kitchens of many American households.

Diet and Cardiovascular Disease

Though the death rate from coronary heart disease has been declining for the past decade, heart attack remains the Number One cause of death in the U.S., killing approximately 560,000 individuals each year. An estimated *1.5 million* people in this country will have heart attacks in the next twelve months; more than one-third of those will be fatal. And there are some 4.6 million people in the U.S. today with *diagnosed* coronary-artery disease. Millions more are almost certainly in varying stages of this disease without yet knowing they have it. Coronary-artery disease is characterized by fatty deposits in the arteries, deposits that restrict and in some cases completely block flow of blood to the heart. (Strokes are caused by similar fatty deposits in arteries leading to the brain.)

Nearly everyone by now has heard that cholesterol and various fats in our diet are somehow involved in heart and blood-vessel diseases. Cholesterol is widely regarded as something "bad." In fact, though, it is absolutely essential for life. Our bodies actually manufacture cholesterol—mainly in the liver and gut—and use it in nearly every cell; it is vital for normal cellular metabolism and for the production of a number of substances, including the sex hormones and other steroids. Only one-fifth of the cholesterol found in our bodies is derived from diet; the rest is made by the body.

So how does cholesterol get us into trouble? The problems begin to arise when too much cholesterol remains in the blood after its vital functions in the body have been performed. An excess may occur because the body produces too much of its own cholesterol (this can be an inherited trait), because too much is entering the body through diet, because cholesterol transport systems (delivering excess back to the liver for breakdown) are defective or because other mechanisms of excreting cholesterol from the body are inadequate.

The term "fat" is a loose one and, in general usage, embraces several types of compounds. Some people refer in this general way to cholesterol as a fat, though it is really a different substance (a steroid) that, however, is found only in products of animal origin and is usually associated with animal fats (including egg yolks). Cholesterol is not the only culprit in cardiovascular disease. There are also neutral fats or triglycerides, found in animal fats, which participate, as well, in clogging the arteries. The "saturated" fats are those of animal origin.

No one any longer disputes the association between elevated serum cholesterol and increased risk of cardiovascular disease. In other words, if you have high concentrations of cholesterol in your blood, you are more likely than someone with lower concentrations to have a heart attack or develop some other manifestation of cardiovascular disease, including stroke. In the famous Framingham Heart Study, it was shown that men with an average 260 milligrams of cholesterol per 100 milliliters of blood were three times as likely to have heart attacks as men with readings below 195 milligrams. The *average* male adult cholesterol level in the U.S. is 210 to 220 milligrams—levels most researchers consider too high.

The issue that has been at the center of a raging controversy for more than two decades now has to do with the effect *diet* has on blood levels of cholesterol and triglycerides. Some studies have shown that healthy individuals are capable of handling high dietary cholesterol intake, breaking it down and excreting it before it can accumulate in the arteries. And some other studies have failed to find a relationship between dietary intake of cholesterol and blood concentrations of the substance. There are formidable difficulties, however, in investigating these issues, and many of these studies have been of very poor design.

The American Heart Association has concluded that the *pre-ponderance* of evidence strongly suggests that diet *does* influence serum cholesterol concentrations; it has accordingly recommended a low-cholesterol/low-saturated-fat diet to help prevent cardiovascular disease. It has, at the same time, recommended replacing some of the saturated fats in the diet with polyunsaturated fats (of the sort found in most vegetable oils), since these have been found to actually have a *lowering* effect on cholesterol.

Epidemiological studies of large population groups have consistently shown a strong association between high dietary cholesterol/saturated-fat intake and cardiovascular disease. Populations that have low saturated-fat intake have a low incidence of these diseases. In addition, there is a great deal of animal research—and some experimental human research—showing that diets high in cholesterol and animal fats lead to narrowing of the arteries. Moreover, by later replacing the high-saturated-fat diet with one low in these fats, the fatty "plaques" that clog the arteries have been seen to partially recede in many experiments.

Significant studies have followed the fates of large numbers of people who have migrated from areas where there is a low incidence of heart disease to areas where there is a high incidence. The Japanese, for example, have relatively little heart disease, compared with Americans; but when Japanese migrate to the U.S. and gradually adopt the American diet, which is high in cholesterol and saturated fats, their incidence of cardiovascular disease goes up very dramatically.

Some continue to argue, though, that other factors, such as smoking, drinking, lack of exercise and stress, may be more responsible for elevated serum cholesterol. Most researchers concede that these other factors play a role, but they are convinced diet is the most important factor. In the animal experiments, nondietary variables often either do not apply or are carefully controlled for, so that the only important difference between experimental and control animals is diet, which nonetheless continues, by itself, to significantly alter the levels of blood lipids and cholesterol.

A very ambitious cholesterol study was recently concluded. Sponsored by the National Heart, Lung and Blood Institute, this ten-year study involved 3,806 men who were placed on dietary and drug regimens designed to lower blood levels of cholesterol. The study lent some of the most powerful support yet forthcoming that reduced dietary intake of cholesterol can lower blood levels of the substance. For every 1 percent reduction in serum cholesterol there is, this study concluded, a 2 percent reduction in the rate of coronary heart disease. Dietary changes at any point in life were found to be beneficial, but the earlier the changes are made the better. Many researchers regard this study as conclusive; its major effect is bound to be a renewed push for low-cholesterol, low-saturated-fat diets.

As you read Part Two of this book you will come across a great many micronutrients, other food supplements and drugs that have been found to have varying effects on cholesterol and lipids in the body. These are as diverse as aspirin and fiber. Recently it has been discovered that there are substances in fatty fish and various other marine animals—of the sort that have been prohibited in most of the low-cholesterol/low-fat diets— that can have potent cholesterol-*lowering* effects—very good news for seafood lovers.

A study some years ago involved feeding human volunteers a pound of shrimp a day for several weeks. Since shrimp contain a lot of cholesterol, researchers expected to see a significant rise in blood levels of cholesterol, as had happened when volunteers were fed large quantities of egg yolks. But no such rise was observed. It was just this sort of puzzling result that helped add fuel to the controversy over the effects of dietary cholesterol on blood levels of cholesterol. If all those shrimp couldn't boost blood levels of cholesterol, what could? Was there really anything to the diet/blood cholesterol theory, after all?

The shrimp mystery has now been cleared up via an exciting discovery. The discovery proceeds in part from epidemiological studies of Greenland Eskimos and other groups that consume large quantities of fatty fish, whale and seal meat (also very high in cholesterol). These groups were found to have very low levels of cholesterol in their blood; they also have a remarkably low incidence of cardiovascular disease. What could account for this? Researchers have now discovered that there are certain fatty acids in these fish and other marine animals that counteract and *lower* cholesterol concentrations in the blood. Unlike cholesterol, these fatty acids are *not* produced by the body and thus can only be obtained through diet or food supplementation.

In one recent study, two groups of individuals were fed a

pound of salmon a day along with salmon oil. One group consisted of healthy people with normal blood lipid/cholesterol concentrations. The other group had abnormally high levels of cholesterol and lipids. The results of the "salmon-a-day" diet were clear-cut. Even in the "normal" group (and many researchers think that what we presently call "normal" could actually stand some improvement with respect to "acceptable" cholesterol blood readings), total cholesterol fell 15 percent and triglycerides fell 40 to 45 percent. Results were even more dramatic in the abnormal group. (For references and further details of these and related studies, see the discussion of "Lipids and Derivatives" in Part Two, especially the analysis of EPA.)

Before leaving fats to consider other dietary factors involved in cardiovascular disease, there are some additional matters you should be aware of. For example, certain vegetable fats are actually "saturated" and thus are not desirable for regular use. These include coconut oil, cocoa butter (the fat of chocolate) and palm oil. These vegetable fats tend to *raise* cholesterol levels.

You should be aware too that even some margarines and shortenings, though advertised as "vegetable," are actually quite high in saturated fats of one type or another. Some are mixtures of different types; check labels upon which the types and amounts of each fat are required to be disclosed. In general, fats that harden when cold are saturated; fats that stay softer or remain liquid are less saturated or are polyunsaturated. Stick margarine has more saturated fats than tub margarine or products that come in squeeze bottles. (Again, check labels; the ratio of polyunsaturated fats to saturates should be 2:1 or better.) Note that most cheeses are high in saturated fats.

The polyunsaturated fats include corn oil, safflower oil, cottonseed oil, soybean oil, sunflower oil, sesame-seed oil. These oils tend to have a cholesterol-lowering effect. (Mono-unsaturated oils, such as olive oil and peanut oil, are neutral as far as cholesterol goes, neither lowering nor raising it.) The lowering effect of the polyunsaturates should not, however, encourage you to eat *all* of these oils you want. Fat, in any form, is still bad in excess; it will contribute to obesity, which, in turn, will predispose you to accelerated aging and disease processes.

The idea, as discussed earlier, should be to eat less fat of all kinds and to reduce in particular the intake of saturated fats.

There are also, in addition to obesity, some distinct dangers associated with excessive intake of polyunsaturated fats. These include increased likelihood of developing gallstones and increased vitamin E requirements. Findings that diets high in polyunsaturates contribute to certain cancers were not confirmed in subsequent studies (*Lancet*, 2:203, 1971). Still, the possibility of cancer is theoretically enhanced by large quantities of polyunsaturates because of their proneness to peroxidation (and thus to the production of free radicals). They require vitamin E to help protect against oxidant damage.

Again, it is advisable to reduce *all* fats in your diet—to about 20 percent of total calories; derive about one-third of those fat calories from saturated fats and the remainder from mono- and polyunsaturated fats.

Other dietary factors to consider in terms of effect on cardiovascular disease are:

CARBOHYDRATES AND FIBER—Total carbohydrate intake has little long-term effect on serum lipid levels in most people. It was believed until recently that high-carbohydrate intake in general raised serum triglyceride levels, but this is not the case (see Connor and Connor, cited above). High intakes of specific types of carbohydrates, principally sugar—as a food additive—may result in mild lipid elevations, while also contributing to obesity and dental caries. Most Americans would benefit from reducing their sugar intake by at least one-half. It is best, in fact, if only about 10 percent of total calories is derived from sucrose—the kind of sugar you add to your foods.

A change in the type of carbohydrate—one favoring complex carbohydrates derived from whole grains, cereals, beans, vegetables and some fruits—has been found to be beneficial in maintaining a healthy cardiovascular system, in part because these carbohydrates provide nutrient-laden calories and extra fiber. The typical American diet is a low-fiber diet consisting of highly refined foods; this low-fiber aspect has now been associated with a number of disorders, including diverticulosis, cancer of the colon, appendicitis, hemorrhoids and varicose veins. High-fiber diets contribute to healthier cardiovascular systems because they tend to be filling and thus discourage overconsumption of fats and cholesterol. In addition, certain types of fiber (see analysis, Part Two) have been shown to control the rate of absorption of glucose in the bloodstream; a reduced rate may have a cardioprotective effect.

PROTEIN—Overall dietary intake of protein has not been shown to affect serum cholesterol/lipid levels. Animal experiments, however, have given indications that some animal proteins, such as casein, *do* raise lipid levels, whereas some vegetable proteins, such as soy protein, lower lipid levels. Human studies have been difficult to control but offer some preliminary evidence that vegetable protein has a cholesterol-lowering effect in humans. De-emphasis of animal protein, in any event, is advised because of the associated animal fats. (See protein recommendations earlier in this chapter.)

ALCOHOL—For those who are not overweight, very moderate alcohol intake may actually be associated with a reduced mortality rate from coronary heart disease. The effects are variable, but, in general, recent studies indicate that one or two drinks a day may lower cholesterol levels; it's a fine line, though, because other studies show that two or more drinks a day will increase heart disease. One beer or one cocktail a day, on average, is probably safe enough—and possibly helpful. Moderation is definitely recommended because, apart from the risks of alcoholism, drinking is associated with certain forms of cancer. (See discussion below.)

SALT—High dietary intake of salt is firmly associated with hypertension (high blood pressure). Hypertension is very much a disease of the Western world. It is almost unheard of in "primitive" societies where salt is not a common food additive. You should work to gradually wean yourself off added salt. Foods may taste bland, even awful, at first without salt, but it is surprising how quickly one adapts to a relatively salt-free diet. Soon it will be the added salt that tastes awful.

Diet and Cancer (And the Search for the Ideal Anticancer Diet)

Evidence that diet is linked to some forms of cancer is extensive and growing rapidly. Some researchers estimate that 90 percent of all cancers are caused by environmental factors. Included in those environmental factors is diet, which some of these authorities believe causes 30 to 60 percent of all human cancers. Epidemiological studies suggest that alterations in diet can prevent many of these cancers, especially those of the stomach and large bowel. They further believe that lesser but still significant prevention can be achieved via dietary modifications with respect to cancers of the lung, breast and endometrium (uterine lining). Effects of dietary change on other cancers remain more speculative.

Since cures for cancer (which currently accounts for about 20 percent of all deaths in the U.S.) have proved elusive in most cases, emphasis has recently shifted to attempts at prevention of the disease. Apart from smoking, which causes fully 25 percent of all fatal cancers in this country, diet is thought to be the next most important factor upon which to focus the preventive effort. Population studies have encouraged researchers to believe that factors at least potentially within our control are at the base of many cancers. Malignancies of the breast, colon and uterus, for example, have consistently been found to be associated with the sort of diet that characterizes affluent societies like our own. Moreover, people living in less affluent, less cancer-prone societies tend to develop these same cancers, and at about the same rate as we do, when they move here and adopt our diet.

Our excessive intake of fat and cholesterol is believed to be the primary dietary culprit. There is some evidence that high-protein diets may also promote some cancers. Data related to cancer and carbohydrates are still very tentative; what evidence exists suggests that refined sugars and starches may increase risk of certain cancers, while complex carbohydrates and dietary fiber may have protective effects. Fortunately, the sort of diet that appears at this time to confer some protection against cancer coincides largely with the diet that has been proposed for protection against cardiovascular disease. This is not surprising since some of the same mechanisms are believed to contribute to both diseases. (For an excellent review of the relevant literature, see *Diet, Nutrition and Cancer*, National Academy Press, Washington, D.C., 1982; also see review by Willett and MacMahon, *New England Journal of Medicine*, 310:663 and 697, 1984.)

In addition to fat, protein and carbohydrates, however, other factors must also be taken into account. Smoking has already been mentioned. Total caloric intake and body weight are factors, as are synthetic and natural mutagens and carcinogens in food, air and water, alcohol, drugs and cosmetics. Let's examine several of the diet-related factors in more detail.

FAT—The human cancers most strongly associated with dietary fats are those of the large bowel and breast. Prostate cancer too has been associated with high-fat intake, though not so strongly as these other cancers. Animal experiments have similarly demonstrated the influence of fat/cholesterol on various cancers, especially those of the breast and colon. Tumor incidence has been seen to rise in several of these studies in direct relation to increased fat intake. Good data are still lacking on which components of fats and cholesterol are the most likely to initiate or promote cancer; what data do exist suggest that the saturated (animal) fats are the ones most often associated with cancer. However, with respect to breast cancer, Enig et al. (*Federation Proceedings, Federation of the American Society for Experimental Biology*, 37:2215, 1978) have noted an association with the sort of trans-fatty acids that are produced when liquid vegetable oils are converted to solid vegetable shortenings and margarine. All of this points up, once again, the need to avoid excessive intake of *any* type of fat.

How fats of all types may contribute to cancer is suggested by studies showing that a number of cancer-causing substances arise as fats and cholesterol are oxidized both before and after they have been ingested. Given the fact that fats account for more than 40 percent of the total calories in the typical American diet, it is not difficult to see how we might be exposed to a significant "load" of carcinogens and to extensive free-radical activity of the sort that accompanies the oxidation and metabolic breakdown of fats.

PROTEIN—It is difficult to separate the effects of dietary fat and protein since they are usually derived, in our diets, from the same animal sources. Protein may have cancer effects independent of the effects of fat, but if so, these have not yet been clearly demonstrated. There are various population studies showing that people who have very high meat intake have higher incidences of cancer (usually of the colon and rectum), but, again, these higher rates could be due to fats, rather than to protein, or to both—or they could be due to the fact that people who fill up on fats and protein often avoid vegetables, fruits and other sources of needed nutrients and fiber.

Greek researchers (*International Journal of Cancer*, 32:1, 1983) reported that 100 Athenians with colorectal cancers had diets that heavily favored meats and largely spurned vegetables, especially cabbage, lettuce, spinach and beets. Comparisons were made with a matching group of 100 Athenians who favored vegetables over meat. The researchers found that those of the high-meat/low-vegetable diet had an *eightfold* increase in risk of getting colorectal cancers as compared with those on the low-meat/high-vegetable diet. Again, it is difficult to sort all of this out, but it seems likely that multiple factors are at play here. High fat appears to be contributing to cancer; high animal protein *might* be, and vegetables, especially those in the cabbage family (see discussion below), have recently been shown to confer some special protection against some cancers.

In the U.S., other studies have shown, the Seventh-Day Adventists, who are largely vegetarians, have only half the overall national colorectal cancer rate. It must be noted, though, that they also tend to avoid alcohol, smoking, coffee and tea. The Seventh-Day Adventists, by the way, have average life expectancies seven years longer than the average non-Adventist.

Despite all the ambiguities, there appears to be at least some weak correlation between high animal-protein intake and cancers of the breast, colon, rectum, prostate, endometrium, pancreas and kidney. In animal studies, the ability of various substances to induce cancer seems to be promoted by protein intake that is two to three times the normal requirement for optimal growth and development. And this ability to cause cancer is *decreased* when animals are given amounts of protein at or below the minimum amount needed for optimal growth.

There are some who believe that Americans, who derive about 15 percent of their total calories from protein, are getting more than they need. But most researchers still think that 15 percent is about right. And, until further data are in, I would have to agree. What needs to be altered is not the amount but the source of protein. We need to get less of our total protein from animal sources and more from vegetable sources, along the lines suggested above in the discussion of diet and cardiovascular disease.

CARBOHYDRATES—The data here are too inconclusive for any but the most tentative pronouncements. There is very preliminary evidence that diets high in refined sugars may contribute to cancer. Complex, unrefined carbohydrates, on the other hand, may actually help protect against some cancers.

DIETARY FIBER—The best available evidence suggests but does not yet prove that dietary fiber protects against some cancers, principally those of the colon and rectum. (See analysis of fiber in Part Two for further details.) One theory is that fiber may dilute fecal constituents that contribute to cancer and that fiber, moreover, speeds the passage of these carcinogens out of the colon and rectum before they can do much damage. The theory is a sensible one, but more work will be required before we can say *for sure* that fiber protects against malignancy.

VEGETABLES—Certain green vegetables, especially those of the cabbage family, deserve special mention. A number of studies (see analysis under Wheatgrass/Barley Grass and Some Other Green Plants in Part Two) have indicated that some green plants appear to contain as yet unidentified substances that may have significant anticancer effects. (See also in Part Two the discussion of vitamin A/beta-carotene and their vegetable sources.)

ALCOHOL AND SMOKING—Alcohol has been associated with cancers of the mouth, esophagus, pharynx and larynx. A weaker association has been made with cancer of the liver. Smoking by itself, as noted above, accounts for a quarter of all cancer deaths in the U.S. Those who regularly smoke two packs of cigarettes a day live eight years *less*, on average, than nonsmokers. (Which is not to say that one pack a day or even half a pack a day gets you off the hook; it doesn't, though the *less* you smoke, the better.) Those who *both* smoke and drink are at even greater risk of getting a number of cancers. There is some evidence that the regular inclusion of green vegetables in the diet reduces *some* of the alcohol-related cancer risks. And there is similarly some evidence that the regular ingestion of carrots and other foods containing beta-carotene may help protect, to some extent, against smoking-induced lung cancers.

TOTAL CALORIC INTAKE/BODY WEIGHT—There is some evidence, though it is not conclusive, that increased caloric intake and obesity are associated with increased cancer risks. (See, for example, Lew and Garfinkel's weight/mortality survey of some 750,000 men and women, *Journal of Chronic Diseases*, 32:563, 1979.) The strongest associations are with cancers of the endometrium (lining of the womb) and gallbladder. There is an association with breast cancer, as well, but it is less strong. Work with animals indicates that those on restricted caloric intake live longer and have fewer cancers than those animals permitted to eat as much as they want. More research is required before the issue is resolved, but for now, at least, it appears that obesity is a risk factor for both cancer and cardiovascular disease.

DIETARY CARCINOGENS (NATURAL AND SYNTHETIC)— Some 3,000 substances are added to food in the United States in the course of processing; another estimated 12,000 chemical substances that are not intended as additives get into food occasionally. The effects of most of these substances on human health—and on cancer in particular—remain unknown. There are laws that say you can't add known carcinogens to food, but even most of the 3,000 intended additives have never been adequately tested for carcinogenicity. In addition, many foods contain *natural* carcinogens or mutagens (substances capable of causing alterations in the genetic program of cells and thus, often, of causing cancer).

New methods of analysis have turned up some surprises in foods we commonly eat. (See *Science*, 221:1256, 1983.) Carcinogenic hydrazines, for example, have been found, as natural constituents, in edible mushrooms. Hydrazines are believed to cause cancer through production of oxygen radicals. Other carcinogens, called furocoumarins, have been found in celery, parsnips, figs and parsley, again as natural constituents. The concentration of these carcinogens appears to increase dramatically in some of these plants when they are diseased. This may be accounted for, in part, by the fact that some of these carcinogens are the plants' natural defenses against bacteria, fungi, insects and other enemies.

Black pepper and oil of sassafras, which has been used in sarsaparilla root beer, contain other carcinogens. So do potatoes when they are bruised or diseased. Chocolate, cocoa powder, fava beans, rhubarb, coffee, oil of mustard and horseradish, cottonseed oil, okra and even alfalfa sprouts have also recently been reported to contain natural carcinogens and/or mutagens.

Biochemist Bruce Ames, author of the *Science* article cited above, estimated that "the human dietary intake of 'nature's pesticides' is likely to be several grams a day—probably at least 10,000 times higher than the dietary intake of man-made pesticides." Whether we're better adapted, however, to cope with "nature's own" remains to be seen.

For now, no one is recommending we stop eating potatoes or celery, though we should try to ensure, whenever possible, that the plants we eat are *fresh* and relatively free from disease. Black pepper and oil of sassafras, on the other hand, are items most of us can probably do easily enough without. Purists will want to scratch chocolate and coffee from their menus as well; even before these new findings came along, neither coffee nor chocolate received good nutritional marks anyway. Heavy coffee drinking, in fact, is linked, in preliminary studies, with cancers of the bladder, ovary, pancreas and large bowel. Mustard and horseradish aren't likely to do much harm unless they become a major part of your diet. As for alfalfa sprouts, it's possible that they, like a lot of green vegetables, also contain *anti*carcinogens, but we don't *know* that yet for sure.

Moldy foods should be avoided. Some of the most potent carcinogens known are molds that sometimes turn up in peanut butter, bread, some cheeses, etc. Foods preserved by salt-curing, salt-pickling or smoking should be avoided too, as these give rise to nitrosamines that are almost certainly carcinogenic in humans.

Burned/browned foods are perhaps the major sources of dietary carcinogens. There are substances in protein that when heated, and especially when browned or burned, become highly mutagenic. Even the brown crusts of bread have been shown to contain substances that damage DNA and appear to be carcinogenic. Dr. Ames estimates that the typical American family is ingesting several grams of these burned or brown protein substances per day. You can find the same kinds of mutagens in the urine of people who consume a meal of fried pork or bacon that you find in the urine of people who smoke cigarettes regularly. This is not to say that the risks are equal, but such comparisons provide a starting point for evaluating relative risks.

Cooking of fats and oils—and especially the *reheating* of oils —increases their rancidity reactions and thus increases free-radical activity and carcinogenic potential. Don't save fats/oils you've used in cooking for reuse or reheating.

If all of the above now has you afraid to take another bite of anything, remember that the body has many ways of combating natural and man-made carcinogens, via, for example, the antioxidants discussed earlier and analyzed in more detail in Part Two. Even then, however, information on dietary carcinogens should be used to help reshape reasonable and useful dietary modifications. By being careful about what and how much we eat, the incidence of many cancers can be decreased, just as cardiovascular disease is already being decreased through dietary change.

Summary: Putting It All Together

The best "long-life" diet that can be devised at the present time calls, in general, for:

1) Sufficient caloric restriction to prevent obesity.
2) Reduction of cholesterol and fats and especially of saturated fats, so that total fat provides no more than 30 or, preferably, 20 percent of total calories.
3) Greater reliance upon vegetable sources of protein and less reliance upon meat (some suggest that we get about 45 percent of our protein from vegetable sources and 55 percent from animal sources).
4) Increased intake of complex carbohydrates and less reliance upon refined sugars and starches; emphasis should be on whole grains and cereals, beans, peas, and other vegetables and fruits. Calories lost from cutting back on fats should be made up for by an increase in carbohydrates of these types.
5) Increased intake of dietary fiber.
6) A sharp reduction of salt intake.
7) Alcohol restriction.
8) No smoking.
9) Liberal use of vegetables, especially those in the cabbage family and those rich in beta-carotene.

10) Avoidance of smoked, salt-pickled, salt-cured foods.
11) Avoidance of charred, burned and, when possible, browned foods.
12) Reduced intake of cooked, heated and reheated fats/oils.
13) Coffee restriction.
14) Avoidance of excessive additives, known/suspected carcinogens.
15) Liberal use of foods containing antioxidants (see subsequent chapters).
16) Micronutrient supplementation (see next chapter and Part Two).

three

MICRONUTRIENTS: "MAGIC BULLETS" IN THE WAR ON AGING?

The "Magic" in Perspective (Swords, Not Bullets, But Sharp Ones)

Do vitamins and minerals do any good? A lot of people obviously think so. As previously noted, in the United States alone consumers are spending more than $3 billion annually on vitamins, minerals and other food supplements. Surveys indicate that half of the national population is taking micronutrient supplements in the belief that diet is inadequate to supply all the nutrients that are needed, in the belief that supplements will help prevent diseases (or improve existing diseases) and that they will boost energy and overall feeling of well-being. Many believe, in addition, that supplements will help delay the effects of aging.

Even some of the more conservative bastions of the "medical establishment" are beginning to take a more yielding, sometimes downright accommodating, line on vitamin/mineral supplementation. A popular magazine, *American Health* (Mar./Apr. 1983, p. 39), interviewed a number of prominent medical researchers and revealed that many of them take various vitamins and minerals, sometimes in doses far exceeding government recommendations. The National Cancer Institute, meanwhile, is actively investigating the possibility of preventing a number of cancers, in part through micronutrient manipulation. The NCI, in fact, has started conducting international conferences devoted entirely to the relationship between micronutrients and cancer prevention. NCI is now actively encouraging researchers to submit proposals for human clinical trials of various micronutrients that are believed or hypothesized to be natural inhibitors of various types of cancer—for testing on both high-risk populations and on healthy populations.

The National Research Council of the National Academy of Sciences in 1982 issued its highly influential report, *Diet, Nutrition and Cancer* (cited previously), demonstrating numerous significant links between both macronutrition (diet as a whole) and various micronutrients and other food supplements/additives. Articles now appear in such circumspect publications as the *Journal of the American Medical Association* reporting the favorable effects of certain supplements in some disorders. Speakers at the American Heart Association meetings now similarly extol the virtues of various vitamins and minerals without undue self-consciousness or apology.

The NCI, in collaboration with the National Heart, Lung and Blood Institute, is joining forces to investigate the effects of a vitamin-A-related substance called beta-carotene (thought to have significant anticancer effects). Harvard Medical School has recruited 20,000 physicians to participate in an ambitious long-term study using beta-carotene. The times are definitely changing. It wasn't very long ago that the medical establishment was almost unified in its insistence that the public needn't worry about vitamins, minerals and other micronutrients because, it was claimed, people were getting all of those they needed in the "great American diet."

Now that same medical establishment is beginning to acknowledge that it is this same "great American diet" that is kill-ing us in record numbers. Not only is this diet a macronutrient disaster (see discussion in the preceding chapter), it is also a micronutrient miser. A number of studies indicate that many Americans, especially the elderly, are deficient in at least one micronutrient and in some cases several, particularly vitamins B_6, C and A, and the minerals magnesium, calcium, iron and zinc.

A number of factors, some of them detailed in the last chap-ter, have conspired to turn our "standard" diet against us. We get entirely too many of our calories from fat and processed carbohydrates. We tend ever more, it seems, toward "fast" or "convenience" foods, which, again, are often made up of nu-trient-short fats, sugars and other overrefined carbohydrates. Freezing, overcooking and overrefining rob food of nutrients and sometimes add potentially dangerous substances to what we eat. We typically end up with an overabundance of calories but not enough nutrients. Many of us get far too many of our total calories from booze, which contains almost nothing of nutrient value. (See *Journal of the American Dietetic Association*, Apr. 1983.)

Meanwhile, as the bad news about our typical diet has been spreading, good news has been cropping up all over the place with respect to the positive effects various micronutrients can have if present, either through diet or supplementation, in ade-quate quantities. So both the bad news and the good news—knowledge, in a word—have joined forces to encourage micro-nutrient supplementation. The quality of that knowledge is steadily improving. We are learning more all the time about how our nutritional requirements change with age and circum-stance.

It is now known, for example, that women can benefit from extra supplementation of various nutrients (see parts Two and Three) for which there may not be as great an indication in men. That goes for women in general; they tend to exhibit more nutritional deficiencies than their male counterparts. Research is yielding information suggesting that women on the birth-con-trol pill, postmenopausal women, pregnant women and nursing mothers all have their own special micronutrient needs.

This is not to say that men don't suffer from nutritional defi-ciencies too, Men who have certain types of infertility can ben-efit from special micronutrient regimens. Certainly smokers and drinkers need some extra supplementation. So, typically, do individuals who are hospitalized, especially for surgery. (Malnutrition in hospitals is widespread; see, for example, *Journal of Bone and Joint Surgery*, Dec. 1982, in which it is reported that 40 percent or more of all surgical patients may suffer from malnutrition while in the hospital—malnutrition sufficient to cause cardiovascular and other disorders.) People on weight-loss diets are others who are at particular risk of developing micronutrient deficiencies. So are people who regularly use various antacids and some other over-the-counter and prescription drugs. Athletes, including runners, joggers, weight lifters, constitute another important subcategory vulnerable to deficiencies. The aged are perhaps the most vulnerable of all. (See Parts Two and Three for supplement information; some specific micronutrient regimens for individual subgroups are provided in Part Three.)

As the nutritional news, both good and bad, has spread, so has the desire for some quick fix, some easy answer. People are looking for the magic bullets that will quickly, if not instantly, vanquish stress, lack of energy, various diseases, aging itself. Not surprisingly, some of the manufacturers of vitamins, minerals and other food supplements have been all too eager to claim that their products *are* those magic bullets.

As you read Part Two of this book, which sorts out all the claims that have been made, both pro and con, you'll discover that there are no magic bullets, although there are some sharp swords we can now wield with considerable success against certain of the major diseases associated with aging. The magic-bullet idea, however, must be set aside for now, for not only is it false, it's also very dangerous. The moment, for example, that a micronutrient is identified as being particularly useful in protecting against lung cancer, many smokers jump to the conclusion that they can now smoke with impunity so long as they take large doses of the nutrient in question. Similarly, a great many people who don't take time to eat well-balanced meals are lulled by the magic-bullet philosophy into thinking they are "all right" so long as they faithfully take their "one-a-day" or their "stress" formula, etc.

Obviously, people who haven't got their macronutrient act together, along the lines suggested in the preceding chapter, *do*, more than most others, need to take micronutrient supplements. But these people should not delude themselves, any more than the smokers should, that taking supplements will make up for everything else. In addition, the magic-bullet approach tends to highlight individual nutrients or other supplements, touting them, individually, as panaceas, cure-alls. This promotes a faddist approach and detracts from the need for a thoughtful, integrated program of micronutrient supplementation.

Why Supplements Should *Help* (Antioxidant Impact on Cancer and Other Age-Related Diseases)

Apart from the fact that millions of us do suffer from nutritional deficiencies (see Part Two for specific evidence), which, logically, should be at least somewhat correctable via supplementation, there is now also a considerable body of knowledge related to the mechanisms by which various of the micronutrients act to defeat some of the underlying causes of disease and aging. In other words, there are both convincing theories and persuasive findings that make it evident that supplementing our diets with various micronutrients *should* favorably affect the aging process.

You will find, as you read Part Two, that many different nutrients act in different, although sometimes only slightly different, ways to achieve their favorable ends. And you should rely upon each individual analysis for an explanation of how any given supplement works or is believed to work. The present discussion is of a more general nature; it focuses upon what is perhaps the most important anti-aging effect of them all, that achieved by the antioxidants.

Let's look first at cancer.

As explained in the preceding chapter, most of the carcinogens to which we are exposed every day generate free radicals, which, in turn, play a part in the accumulation of lipofuscin (the so-called "age pigment"), in the production of cross-links and in the activity of other factors that, cumulatively, diminish or destroy the ability of individual cells to function properly.

Free radicals have a special affinity for cell membranes and fatty acids; they tend to oxidize and hence hasten the rancidification of fats, giving rise to chemicals that themselves do further damage to cells. The end product of all this is often disease, frequently cancer, but also heart disease, senility and so on.

It has been hypothesized that 80 to 90 percent of all cancers are due to environmental factors. Smoking, which produces free radicals, is certainly one of the most significant of these factors. The high fat content of our diets appears to be one of the other major factors, especially with respect to colon and breast cancers, which (along with lung cancer) account for *half* of all cancer deaths in the U.S. The fat situation is worth examining here, for it helps illustrate how free radicals do their damage and how antioxidant supplements can help prevent some of that damage.

Some 40 percent of the calories we consume daily in the U.S. are derived, on average, from fat. A significant amount of this is oxidized fat—the sort capable of inflicting a lot of free-radical damage. Cooking in particular can oxidize unsaturated fatty acids (of the sort found in most vegetable oils) and cholesterol (found in association with animal fats), and out of this oxidation process there arise a number of substances that have been identified as carcinogens. The DNA program of the cells is easily damaged by these carcinogens and free radicals. This damage promotes accelerated aging, mutation and malignancy.

Fortunately, we are not without defenses against these free-radical attacks. Among the dietary antioxidant defenses are:

VITAMIN E—This vitamin is particularly important in protecting the lipid (fatty acid) membranes; it is protective against free-radical-generating substances that have been linked to both cancer and cardiovascular disease. In addition, Dr. Ames (cited earlier) notes that "vitamin E markedly increases the endurance of rats during heavy exercise, which causes extensive oxygen radical damage to tissues."

BETA-CAROTENE—This vitamin-A-related substance (much less toxic in large doses than the vitamin itself) has been shown to be a powerful antioxidant, putting out the "fires" that do the damage to cells and lipid membranes. Protective effects have been reported in smokers, and definite anticancer effects have been observed in lab animals.

SELENIUM—Dr. Ames observes that this mineral "significantly inhibits the induction of skin, liver, colon and mammary tumors in experimental animals." There is growing epidemiological evidence that low selenium intake is a risk factor for cancer in humans. Selenium is essential for the activity of one of the most important of all the free-radical-neutralizing enzymes—glutathione peroxidase.

ASCORBIC ACID (VITAMIN C)—This is another very important antioxidant that has been shown to have anticancer effects in certain lab animals. There is some evidence that it may protect against precancerous cervical dysplasia in humans.

Cancer is not the only disease in which free radicals play an important role. The oxidation of fat appears to contribute to heart disease as well, and many of the antioxidants, especially selenium and vitamin E, appear to provide some protection against some of the root causes of heart disease. It is possible, in fact, to postulate a free-radical mechanism at the root of all degenerative processes, including those of the brain, nervous and reproductive systems. "The brain," Dr. Ames notes, "uses 20 percent of the oxygen consumed by man and contains an appreciable amount of unsaturated fat." This creates a potentially risky situation—one of, to put it inelegantly, rancid fat in the brain. Likely consequences are various brain abnormalities and senile dementia.

As exciting as the emerging antioxidants are, they are not the whole story. Micronutrients act in a diversity of ways—as will be evident when you read Part Two—to help prevent disease and retard aging.

PART TWO

ANTI-AGING NUTRIENTS:

*What They Can
and Can't Do*

SIGNIFICANT DISCOVERIES

What follows is an introductory sampling of some of the promising and important findings about individual micronutrients and other food supplements that are analyzed in detail in the following chapters. Some of these findings have been emerging for years, gathering confirmation, but may only now be leaving the laboratory to enter public consciousness. Some others are newer and will require further scrutiny before they are widely accepted.

You will note, as you read this sampling, and more specifically as you study the rest of Part Two, that micronutrients seem to have favorable effects on almost all of the degenerative processes related to aging—cancer, heart-and-circulatory disorders, arthritis and autoimmune diseases, brain disorders and some forms of senility, bone and joint diseases, diabetes and immune-related diseases. Some of the results have been more dramatic than others; each nutrient must be studied and evaluated on its own merits, as it is in subsequent chapters.

The following is merely a sampling and not a comprehensive summary of significant findings, arranged by nutrient categories (i.e., vitamins, minerals, amino acids, etc.). If you are interested in all the relevant findings with respect to a specific disease or disorder, such as arthritis, consult the index to help you find the information you seek in the various sections in Part Two. *Before taking any supplements, review the detailed analyses and recommendations in the following chapters of Part Two. Studies alluded to below will be found in these chapters.* Some important negative, as well as positive, findings are included in the following sampling, but further details appear later in Part Two.

Vitamins

VITAMIN A/BETA-CAROTENE—A great deal of attention has recently been focused on vitamin A and one of its precursors, beta-carotene, as possible anticancer substances. There are several epidemiological studies that suggest that diets rich in these nutrients exert a protective effect against many major forms of cancer, including lung cancer. One recent human study failed to find this protective effect, but the researchers involved acknowledged a number of factors that may have biased their results, which, for example, were the product of a single measurement of the blood carotenoid levels and may thus not have truly reflected long-range dietary intake (see Willett et al. *New England Journal of Medicine*, 310:430, 1984). The preponderance of evidence continues to suggest that beta-carotene, which is a potent neutralizer of free radicals, has cancer-preventive properties, at least with respect to some cancers and in some subgroups of the population.

NIACIN (VITAMIN B₃)—The most significant niacin findings indicate that this nutrient, in the form of nicotinic acid, can significantly reduce cholesterol levels and the recurrence rate for heart attacks. Some research even suggests that niacin may be capable of reversing the process of atherosclerosis (narrowing and hardening of the arteries). Some researchers have concluded that niacin is the most effective agent presently available for lowering both cholesterol and triglycerides.

VITAMIN B₆—Excessive megadoses of this vitamin have recently been shown to be dangerous—capable of producing serious nerve damage. In moderation, however, vitamin B_6—pyridox-ine—plays many useful roles in the body. It acts on neurotrans-mitters in the brain and has been shown to vanquish certain types of seizures and convulsions in infants. There are prelimi-nary reports that it is effective in achieving relief from premen-strual tension and that it may be therapeutic in some forms of diabetes. Very recent work, also preliminary, suggests that B_6 may play some favorable role in boosting immunity and in the inhibition of certain cancers, including melanoma (a usually deadly form of skin cancer).

PANTOTHENIC ACID—Part of the vitamin B complex, panto-thenic acid has recently been shown to have some possible fa-vorable effects in the treatment of rheumatoid arthritis. In ani-mal experiments, large doses of pantothenic acid have produced longer survival times under adverse conditions.

VITAMIN C—Also known as ascorbic acid, vitamin C is probably the best known of all the micronutrients, insofar as the public is concerned. Vitamin C is an established antioxidant in the human body. Claims that it can prevent human cancers remain controversial and unresolved. One major recent study, how-ever, indicates that ascorbic acid may protect women from cer-vical dysplasia, a condition that, unchecked, may lead to cancer of the cervix. As an antioxidant, vitamin C has been shown many times to be capable of blocking the formation in the human body of various cancer-causing substances, principally the nitrosamines, which many of us are exposed to in food and water daily. There is evidence that vitamin C favorably affects various mechanisms of the immune system though its ability to prevent or cure the common cold has not been established.

Several studies suggest that vitamin C can inhibit the forma-tion of potentially life-threatening blood clots though this has not been conclusively proved. Other research indicates vitamin C speeds wound healing, helps overcome certain forms of male infertility, may be useful in some forms of asthma, and may protect against some of the damage of smoking and other pol-lutants.

VITAMIN E—There is growing evidence that the role vitamin E plays in human health is considerably more significant than many researchers believed. A great deal of needed information about this nutrient still eludes us, however, and moderation is recommended in terms of supplementation. Up until recently, most of the claims made for vitamin E related to protective effects against cardiovascular disease. Most of these claims have *not* been substantiated. An exception has to do with intermittent claudication, a narrowing of the arteries in the legs. Here, vitamin E supplementation has had favorable effects in humans. And there is growing evidence that vitamin E can help inhibit the formation of potentially lethal blood clots. Vitamin E is a recognized antioxidant and, in that capacity, may help protect us against some forms of pollution. It *may*, especially in collaboration with the mineral selenium, have some anticancer effects, but these remain to be convincingly demonstrated. There is some recent, promising research indicating that supplemental vitamin E is useful in the treatment of mammary dysplasia (abnormal growth of cells in the breast). Claims of immune-boosting properties are being investigated.

Minerals

CALCIUM—A number of subgroups have been found to be at special risk of calcium deficiency, including the aged, postmenopausal women, people on various types of diets, including high-fiber diets, pregnant women, regular users of antacids containing aluminum, heavy users of alcohol, etc. The most significant contribution of calcium supplementation appears to be the prevention of osteoporosis, which afflicts literally millions of Americans and is characterized by diminished bone mass and a tendency to bone fracture, usually increasing with age. There is some emerging, preliminary evidence that calcium may be useful in the treatment of high blood pressure.

CHROMIUM (AND GLUCOSE TOLERANCE FACTOR)—Impaired glucose tolerance appears to increase with age. Studies have shown that this tolerance improves in elderly subjects when diet is supplemented with chromium. Younger persons may derive benefits from chromium, as well. The impact on diabetes, however, remains to be explored.

COPPER—Copper has antioxidant functions that may be of particular importance in the human body. There is a growing body of animal and experimental data suggesting that copper may have anticancer effects, though these remain to be demonstrated in humans. These findings—and others suggestive of effects protective against cardiovascular disease—deserve thorough follow-up. There is good evidence that copper plays an anti-inflammatory role in the body and may be useful in the treatment of some forms of arthritis—though usually in the form of pharmaceutical complexes containing copper.

IRON—Iron is the treatment of choice for iron-deficiency anemia, though not for pernicious anemia. Iron, like copper, has antioxidant properties. There is evidence that iron plays important roles in cellular immunity and bacterial killing. It is also involved in the production of energy, and deficiencies may, apart from the effects of any anemia, result in decreased physical endurance. Both skeletal and cardiac muscular performance require sufficient amounts of iron for optimal efficiency. There is gathering evidence that iron deficiencies may contribute to learning and behavioral disorders.

MAGNESIUM—There are signs that marginal magnesium deficiency may be commonplace, especially among a number of subgroups, including athletes and others who exercise regularly and strenuously, among the elderly, pregnant women, dieters and others. The most significant findings indicate that magnesium is protective against some forms of cardiovascular disease. Magnesium has to be in the proper balance with calcium; when it is not, a number of adverse events can occur, predisposing to heart-tissue damage and heart attack. It has been convincingly demonstrated that magnesium deficiency predisposes humans to potentially fatal cardiac dysrhythmias (abnormal cardiac rhythms). There is some evidence that magnesium supplements may be useful in the management of high blood pressure.

MANGANESE—Manganese can be either antioxidant or prooxidant, depending upon form. Fortunately, it appears to exist in the antioxidant form in the brain and thus helps protect against degenerative neurological diseases.

MOLYBDENUM—It was recently established that a pervasive molybdenum deficiency in the Lin Xian region of China was responsible for the world's highest incidence of esophageal cancer. Now, with the addition of this mineral to the soil, the incidence of this particular cancer appears to be declining in that region of China for the first time in more than two thousand years. There is also experimental evidence that molybdenum can prevent some cancer by inhibiting the formation of various chemical carcinogens.

SELENIUM—This mineral is probably exciting more research interest at the present time than any other micronutrient. It is an important antioxidant and appears to be capable of reducing the incidence of a variety of cancers. Epidemiological studies show a higher incidence of several cancers in areas where the soil is low in selenium than in areas where the soil is rich in this element. High Japanese selenium intake has been credited with the low incidence of breast cancer in Japan. The National Academy of Sciences has concluded that "a large accumulation of evidence indicates that supplementation of the diet or drinking water with selenium protects against tumors induced by a variety of chemical carcinogens and at least one viral agent." Selenium may have antitumor as well as cancer-preventive effects, but this is not as well established. There is some possibility that selenium helps other nutrients, such as vitamin E, exert anti-cancer effects. There is growing evidence that selenium has immunostimulant effects and may thus help ward off infection.

Selenium appears, in addition, to have potentially important effects that are protective against cardiovascular disease. Epidemiological studies show that the so-called "stroke belt" of the United States, an area in the southeast U.S., is characterized by very low selenium content in the soil. This area has the highest stroke rate in the country and also has a very high heart-disease rate. Selenium supplementation alone, and in combination with vitamin E, has yielded promising results in some individuals suffering from various cardiovascular disorders.

Selenium is, however, highly toxic in other than minute doses. Fortunately only small doses are needed.

ZINC—Zinc is of enormous importance in human health, Its many vital roles in the human body are only now beginning to be appreciated. Zinc is emerging, in particular, as a major factor in maintenance of the immune system. The decline of the immune system with age, it now appears, can be at least partially reversed with adequate zinc supplementation. Zinc deficiencies appear to be far more widespread than once imagined. Zinc supplements have been shown to increase the number of circulating T-lymphocytes, which fight infection; it has also been shown to improve antibody response. Zinc accelerates wound healing and is useful in the treatment of some forms of infertility. Findings with respect to cancer continue contradictory. Further research is indicated to clarify zinc's potential beneficial effects in some cancers. Preliminary findings that zinc supplementation may be useful in some diabetics and sufferers of rheumatoid arthritis are equally deserving of follow-up.

Amino Acids

L-ARGININE—Arginine has a stimulating effect on human growth hormone and has been promoted as a muscle-building, fat-burning nutrient. Serious study is only beginning to investigate these claims. Arginine shows some signs of speeding wound healing and stimulating the immune system. There are preliminary animal data suggestive of antitumor effects.

L-CYSTEINE—Extended life-spans have been reported in guinea pigs injected with this amino acid, which is believed to have antioxidant effects. Cysteine has also been reported effective in protecting against certain toxic substances and in promoting DNA repair.

L-LYSINE—Claims that lysine can inhibit herpes virus have not been substantiated.

TAURINE—Oral taurine supplementation has been shown, in preliminary work, to be of some benefit as an anticonvulsant in human epilepsy.

TYROSINE—There are some indications that tyrosine may be useful in the treatment of some forms of mental depression. This finding may be of some significance, especially in view of the side effects of the currently used antidepressants, but more work will have to be done in order to confirm this.

TRYPTOPHAN—There is preliminary evidence that this amino acid may have sedative and pain-killing effects.

Nucleic Acids and Derivatives

DNA AND RNA—Oral DNA/RNA supplements are almost certainly worthless; they are destroyed in the digestive system before they reach target tissues. Injectable forms have yielded mixed results, with a few researchers claiming anti-aging effects and significantly extended life-spans in lab animals. A synthetic nucleic acid called PolyA/Poly U has been found to significantly increase the survival time of women who had been operated on for breast cancers. Animal work has lent further credibility to claims that this substance, also given via injection, has immune-stimulating effects.

ADENOSINE—Of possible use in some forms of heart and nerve diseases.

INOSINE—A derivative of inosine has been reported to be effective against certain viral infections.

OROTATE—There is some early indication that orotate may be of use in the treatment of congestive heart failure and the protection of heart muscle.

Lipids and Derivatives

CHOLINE/LECITHIN—Intravenous choline has been shown to lower blood pressure in humans; mixed results have been obtained with *oral* choline/lecithin. There is some evidence that choline/lecithin influence certain of the brain's neurotransmitters and may improve short-term memory in some individuals. There is preliminary evidence that lecithin can improve the condition of patients suffering from *advanced* Alzheimer's disease while *worsening* the condition of those with early Alzheimer's. Lecithin has shown some effectiveness in the treatment of a serious neurological disorder called tardive dyskinesia, which is sometimes a side effect of major tranquilizing drugs.

EPA (FISH OILS)—EPA is a long-chain fatty acid that affects production of prostaglandins, a family of hormonelike substances that have far-reaching effects in the body. Many ocean fish are particularly rich in EPA, and those, such as the Greenland Eskimos, whose diets are rich in fish, seal and whale meat have a very low incidence of heart attack and other manifestations of cardiovascular disease. EPA, several studies indicate, protects against heart disease through prostaglandin activities that, among other things, inhibit blood clots. EPA also appears to lower blood levels of cholesterol and triglycerides.

GLA (AND OIL OF EVENING PRIMROSE)—Oil of evening primrose has become a popular food supplement. It is rich in gamma-linolenic acid (GLA). Like EPA, GLA is supposed to protect against cardiovascular disease, but the evidence here is not nearly so strong. Well-controlled studies still remain to be done.

MYO-INOSITOL—There is evidence that inositol may have some cardioprotective effects in animals, but this has not yet been demonstrated in humans. There is growing evidence that inositol may help protect against one of the major complications of diabetes, peripheral neuropathy, a serious form of nerve disease.

Other Supplements

L-CARNITINE—This substance has been shown to be protective against some forms of cardiovascular disease. It has been shown to be capable of raising blood levels of high-density lipoprotein (HDL) cholesterol. HDL is believed to have a *protective* effect against coronary heart disease. (It is often referred to as "the good cholesterol.") Claims that carnitine can help build muscle and increase stamina have not been proved. The hypothesis that carnitine may be an aid in dieting has some theoretical merit and is worthy of investigation.

DIETARY FIBER—A high-fiber diet is now the treatment of choice for diverticular disease of the colon. Claims that high-fiber diet protects against cancers of the colon and rectum are unproved, though epidemiological evidence suggests this is the case. High-fiber diet is also believed to be useful in the management of diabetes and in lowering serum cholesterol. Fiber's usefulness in weight-reduction diets has been suggested but not proved.

GARLIC—Several studies have shown that garlic can significantly lower those elements of cholesterol that are associated with heart disease. (*Onions* have exhibited some similar, though not so well documented, effects.) Claims that garlic can inhibit some cancers, increase energy and fight infection have not been well substantiated, though there are preliminary studies showing these favorable effects.

GINSENG—This popular medicinal plant is neither worthless nor innocuous as various individuals have claimed. Heavy use has been reported to lead to a "ginseng abuse syndrome," which can result in, among other things, elevated blood pressure, skin eruptions and diarrhea. Soviet researchers have claimed that ginseng is a mood elevator, an immune stimulator and an energy booster. Claims that it is a sexual aphrodisiac remain entirely anecdotal.

PANGAMIC ACID ("VITAMIN B$_{15}$")—This substance is supposed to retard aging and be a virtual panacea. Unfortunately, these claims have not been substantiated. Worse, there has been mislabeling with respect to some of the pangamic-acid products, and some of them have been found to contain potential cancer-causing substances.

SUPEROXIDE DISMUTASE (SOD)—Oral SOD supplements are being touted as super antioxidants and anti-aging substances. In fact, however, these oral supplements are worthless. Oral SOD is destroyed in the digestive tract before it reaches target tissues. Claims that *oral SOD* is useful against arthritis and cancer are completely without any basis in fact. The *injectable* version of bovine copper-zinc SOD (known as Orgotein) has been reported useful in some cases of rheumatoid arthritis. And, in animal experiments, involving transplanted cancers, *injected* SOD increased survival times.

WHEATGRASS/BARLEY GRASS/OTHER GREEN PLANTS—As yet unidentified substances in wheatgrass, barley grass and certain green vegetables (especially those in the cabbage family, including broccoli and Brussels sprouts) are apparently exerting significant anticancer effects, according to a number of studies. These green plants are coming under increasing scrutiny.

MISCELLANEOUS OTHER SUPPLEMENTS—*Acidophilus (yogurt)* is now often recommended by physicians to help patients maintain intestinal and vaginal ecological balances, especially when on antibiotics; *aloe vera* contains anti-inflammatory substances that could account for some of its alleged benefits in accelerating the healing of burns and other skin irritations; there is no evidence at this time that *bee pollen* is useful in any human ailment; the *bioflavonoids* do not, contrary to claims, protect vitamin C or enhance the body's ability to utilize vitamin C, but there is still evidence worthy of further investigation that bioflavonoids may help protect capillaries in rare individuals with bioflavonoid deficiencies; *brewer's yeast* varies enormously from source to source, and the therapeutic claims that have been made for it have not been substantiated; *capsicum (hot pepper)* has recently been shown to have a favorable effect on blood-clotting disease, and its regular use may help prevent blood clots; *coenzyme Q*, in preliminary studies, has shown some ability to enhance the pumping capability of the heart muscle; *glandulars* are worthless; *royal jelly*, like pantothenic acid, has shown some efficacy in the treatment of rheumatoid arthritis and is deserving of further investigation; *spirulina*, despite a multitude of claims made for it, has not been demonstrated to be of any value; *wheat germ, wheat-germ oil* and *octacosanol* are without demonstrated merit, other than to provide some vitamin E.

Pharmaceuticals/ Chemicals

ASPIRIN—Several studies have now suggested, though not yet proved, that aspirin can help prevent the recurrence of heart attacks—by helping to prevent blood clots. An excellent, recent study showed a very substantial reduction in heart attacks among a certain class of heart patients who received aspirin, as compared with a similar set of heart patients who did not get aspirin.

BHA AND BHT—It has recently been claimed that these antioxidants can extend life-span, kill or inactivate herpes viruses and combat cancer. Unfortunately, none of these things has been demonstrated in humans. The use of these synthetic substances, moreover, may pose serious perils. There is some evidence that BHT can actually *promote* certain types of cancer.

DEANER (DMAE)—This is another "miracle" substance, according to the claims, that is supposed to extend life-span. There is some evidence that this drug is useful in certain disorders of the nervous system; there is no evidence that it is a general life extender. In fact, one recent experiment with this substance showed that animals treated with it actually had *shorter* life-spans than control animals that did not get the drug.

DHEA—This hormone has suddenly become a hot property in the supplement supermarket. It is supposed to promote weight loss, extend life-span and fight cancer. None of this has been demonstrated in humans. Some animal studies, however, indicate that this steroid hormone may, at least in those animals tested, inhibit some forms of cancer and promote some measure of weight loss. Adverse side effects may result from use of this substance. More research is needed.

DMSO—This substance, originally used as an industrial solvent, is now often used topically to treat sprains, bruises and arthritis. The FDA has approved *one* use of DMSO—for the treatment of interstitial cystitis, a fibrosis of the bladder wall. Other studies are ongoing to test the effects of DMSO on various cancers, in skin, nerve and autoimmune diseases. Some of the early findings have been promising but require confirmation.

L-DOPA—The suggestion that even healthy people might benefit from regular use of L-dopa, a prescription drug, is potentially dangerous and is not supported by the available evidence. There is one experiment in which life-spans of mice given L-dopa were extended; this study deserves follow-up but does not justify claims that L-dopa is a human life extender. L-dopa has been used with some success in the treatment of Parkinson's disease.

No one should use this drug, which can have potent adverse side effects, without a doctor's supervision.

GEROVITAL H3 (GH3)—There is no scientific support for the claim that GH3 extends human life-span or retards aging. The claim that it is an antidepressant similarly lacks scientific support and, in fact, has been explicitly contradicted by the best available evidence.

HYDERGINE—This drug—widely being touted as a powerful anti-aging substance—has shown promise in the treatment of chronic senile cerebral insufficiency, reportedly improving mood, memory and cognition. Whether it will eventually be found useful in *preventing* some forms of senile dementia remains to be seen.

Let us proceed now to a more thorough analysis of nearly all the nutrients, supplements and other substances for which anti-aging claims have been made. But first, one important point.

A Note on the "RDAs"

The abbreviation "RDA," which you will find frequently in this part of the book, signifies "Recommended Dietary Allowance" or "Recommended Daily Allowance" for the nutrients for which such "allowances" have been established. In the United States there are two organizations that establish RDAs: the Food and Nutrition Board of the National Academy of Sciences and the Food and Drug Administration (FDA). The former organization came out with its most recent RDAs in 1980 and the latter organization in 1979. There are some differences in amounts recommended by the two organizations, but overall they are quite similar. The RDAs that you will find listed on the labels of vitamins and mineral products are those set by the FDA. These are often referred to as "U.S. RDA."

The RDAs are the levels of the essential nutrients considered, in the judgment of these two organizations, to be *adequate* to meet the nutritional needs of *healthy* individuals. No evident vitamin and mineral deficiencies have been observed in healthy people eating diets that provide the RDAs for the various essential nutrients.

Optimal dietary allowances for *optimal* health and *maximum* longevity, on the other hand, have not yet been determined by any federal agency. There is growing evidence that micronutrient intake (of, for example, beta-carotene, calcium, magnesium, selenium) in amounts *higher* than the RDAs may be protective against various diseases of aging, such as cardiovascular disease, cancer and bone disease. Read each analysis in this part of the book carefully, however, before exceeding the RDAs.

four

VITAMINS

Vitamins are a group of chemically unrelated organic (carbon-containing) nutrients that are essential in small quantities for normal metabolism, growth and physical well-being. These nutrients must be obtained through diet since they are either not synthesized in our bodies or are synthesized in inadequate amounts. Our bodies use vitamins to make substances that are vital participants in many of the chemical reactions in our cells, reactions essential for the proper functioning of cells.

Vitamins are traditionally divided into two categories: the fat-soluble vitamins, which can be stored in the body, and the water-soluble vitamins, which are not stored in significant quantities. Some vitamins are fundamental participants in the energy-producing reactions of our bodies. Vitamins themselves, however, are insignificant sources of biological energy.

The fat-soluble vitamins are vitamins A, D, E and K. Vitamin D is derived both from dietary sources and from reactions occurring in sun-exposed skin. The active forms of most vitamins, that is, the substances formed within our cells from dietary vitamins, participate in cellular metabolism (chemical reactions of the cell) as cofactors for the enzymes that are biological catalysts. In contrast, the active form of vitamin D is a hormone important for the regulation of the body's calcium and the production of white blood cells. Vitamin K is derived from dietary sources and also is produced by some of the bacteria residing in our intestines.

The water-soluble vitamins comprise the B vitamins and vitamin C (ascorbic acid). The B vitamins essential for humans are: B_1, or thiamine; B_2, or riboflavin; niacin, which includes both nicotinic acid and nicotinamide; B_6, which encompasses pyridoxine, pyridoxal and pyridoxamine; B_{12}, or cobalamin; folic acid; pantothenic acid; and biotin.

The chemical structures of all of the vitamins essential to man are now known, and whether one consumes a natural or synthetic version of a vitamin, the active principle is identical.

There are other substances that are occasionally considered to be essential vitamins for humans; their vitamin status, however, has not actually been established. These substances include: choline; lipoic acid; *para*-aminobenzoic acid (PABA); inositol; coenzyme Q, or ubiquinone; bioflavonoids; and carnitine. It has been established that some of these substances do in fact have vitamin activity in some animals other than humans.

Although many biochemical and physiological roles for the vitamins are already known, there is much that we do not understand about them. It is often difficult to reconcile deficiency states of some of the vitamins with their known biochemical functions. It is anticipated that the vitamins will continue to be a rich area for both basic and clinical investigation and that new roles for known vitamins will be discovered. And there may be vitamins that we are not yet aware of.

Although consumption of the so-called "well-balanced diet" is still thought by many to supply all the vitamins we need in quantities sufficient for the maintenance of good health, there are certain situations that place people at an increased risk for vitamin-insufficiency states. Among those at risk are people on low-calorie diets, alcoholics, pregnant women, the elderly in general, surgical patients, users of certain medications and strict vegetarians. Vitamin supplementation is prudent in those and other cases that will be identified in subsequent chapters.

Recently there has been an increasing tendency to use

"megadose" quantities (greater than ten times the RDA) of certain vitamins for several reasons: to help with the stress of daily life, to protect against colds, to increase sexual prowess, etc. Evidence for and against megadosing will be presented in the analyses of each of the vitamins. There are defined indications for the use of megadose vitamins as pharmaceutical agents in the treatment of certain pathological conditions, but megadosing in these situations requires a physician's supervision. These conditions include: the use of megadose nicotinic acid to lower blood cholesterol levels; the treatment of certain skin disorders with vitamin A and synthetic vitamin A derivatives; the use of vitamin B_6 to prevent seizures if one takes an overdose of INH, a drug used for the treatment of tuberculosis.

Evidence is gradually accumulating that even well-fed individuals can profit—in terms of optimizing health—by taking vitamin supplements in prudent amounts. In addition to their role in metabolism, certain vitamins are antioxidants and as such protect against toxic oxygen damage. This protection, I believe, helps establish a preventive role for vitamins with respect to a number of degenerative diseases.

Vitamin A/ Beta-Carotene

I. Overview

When it comes to grabbing the headlines these days there's no nutrient that can compete with vitamin A. A couple of examples: "Low Vitamin A Intake Associated with Cancer" (San Francisco *Chronicle*, Oct. 6, 1982); "The Number One Anti-Cancer Vitamin" (*Prevention*, June 1983). And it isn't just the nutritional "true believers" who are beating the drums for vitamin A; scientific papers on the subject are appearing at a prodigious rate, and some of the country's most circumspect cancer researchers are urging us to get out there and eat those carrots (and other foods rich in this vitamin). They are being joined by the National Research Council and the National Cancer Institute, among others. Carrot fever is abroad in the land.

So what's up, doc? Should we all turn into Bugs Bunnies, or are carrots strictly for rabbits? There's no question about vitamin A being essential for human health; that is now clearly established. It is available to us either as preformed vitamin A (technically known as retinol or retinyl esters), found in some of the meats and animal products we eat, or as provitamin A (precursor substances, such as beta-carotene, which are partially converted to vitamin A once inside the body), found in carrots, sweet potatoes, and several other vegetables and fruits. It is beta-carotene that imparts the yellow color to many of these plant foods.

Vitamin A is essential for, among other things, vision (especially night vision), regulation of cell development and for reproduction. Vitamin A deficiencies often result in alterations in skin and mucous membranes that resemble precancerous conditions. This observation has helped stimulate research on vitamin A as a possible anticancer agent or preventive.

What is most encouraging is that all the vitamin A substances appear to afford some protection against cancer-causing agents. Carotenoids, such as beta-carotene, have been shown to have anti-cancer effects in mice and rats and may have such effects in humans as well (*Science*, 221:1256, 1983). The Department of Medicine at Harvard is presently conducting a randomized, placebo-controlled trial of beta-carotene using as subjects a large number of U.S. physicians. The aim is to see if 30 milligrams (the equivalent of 50,000 IUs) of beta-carotene daily can significantly reduce the incidence of a number of human cancers.

Although high doses of preformed vitamin A are associated with various toxic effects, beta-carotene has exhibited very low toxicity. No toxicity was observed in patients using high daily doses of beta-carotene (300 milligrams or 500,000 IUs) for prolonged periods (*Archives of Dermatology*, 113:1229, 1977). Although neither supplementary preformed vitamin A nor beta-carotene appreciably affects blood levels of vitamin A, supplementary beta-carotene *does* significantly raise blood carotenoid levels (*American Journal of Clinical Nutrition*, 38:559, 1983). Some epidemiological studies have found that higher blood levels of retinols or carotenoids are associated with lower risk of various cancers. Beta-carotene probably exerts its protective effects at the tissue level, serving as a trap for a very toxic form of di-oxygen called singlet oxygen. One group of researchers (*Nature*, 290:201, 1981) has called beta-carotene "the most efficient quencher of singlet oxygen thus far discovered."

Research indicates that vitamin A and its analogues may also have favorable effects on the immune system.

In general, results to date suggest that vitamin A and beta-carotene will play important roles in the effort to improve the quality of and prolong the span of human life. But there are a couple of dangers inherent in these optimistic results. Already some people are talking about using vitamin A supplements *in place of* stricter toxic-chemical safety standards or as an excuse for *lowering* those standards. Others have begun to argue that with beta-carotene supplements the dangers of smoking are reduced. The vitamin A family may, in fact, protect against some of the ravages of smoking and the toxic chemicals we come in contact with, but proof of this is still lacking; protection when and if it is demonstrated will almost certainly be only partial. If we develop something that offers some protection, and for that reason decide we can tolerate more of whatever it is we need protection from, then we will have taken one step forward and one step backward, with no resulting progress.

II. Claims

POSITIVE:
1) Has anticancer effects; 2) speeds healing and fights infections; 3) improves vision; 4) fights skin diseases.

NEGATIVE:
1) Highly toxic; 2) may cause birth defects if taken during pregnancy; 3) may cause bone disease among those with chronic kidney failure.

III. Evidence

RELATED TO POSITIVE CLAIMS:

1) Has anticancer effects—A number of population studies suggest that vitamin A exerts anticancer effects. Bjelke (*International Journal of Cancer*, 15:561, 1975) studied the smoking and eating habits of more than 8,000 Norwegian men over a period of five years. Among the smokers, he observed a significantly increased risk of lung cancer among men with the lowest beta-carotene intake. Shekelle and co-workers (*Lancet*, 2:1185, 1981), in a nineteen-year study of nearly 2,000 men in Chicago, made a similar finding; smokers with the lowest intake of beta-carotene were several times more likely to develop lung cancer than

smokers with the highest intake of beta-carotene. No association was found in this study, however, between lung cancer and
retinol (the preformed variety of vitamin A) intake.

Many other researchers have shown results suggestive of cancer-protective effects of beta-carotene related to numerous
human cancers, including the bladder (*Journal of the National
Cancer Institute*, 62:1435, 1979), the larynx (*American Journal
of Epidemiology*, 113:675, 1981), the esophagus (*Nutrition and
Cancer*, 2:143, 1981), the stomach (H. H. Hiatt et al., eds.,
*Origins of Human Cancer, Book A: Incidence of Cancer in Hu-
mans*, Cold Spring Harbor Laboratory, Cold Spring Harbor,
N.Y., 1977, p. 55), the colon/rectum (*Aktuelle Ernahrungsme-
dizin*, 2:10, 1978), the prostate (K. Magnus, ed., *Trends in Can-
cer Incidence*, Hemisphere Publishing Corp., Washington, New
York, London, 1982).

Intriguing though these epidemiological studies are, they do
not *prove*, as Peto and co-workers point out in perhaps the most
important review article yet published on beta-carotene and
cancer (*Nature*, 290:201, 1981), an anticancer effect. It is possible, for example, that people who eat foods high in beta-carotene (mainly vegetables) tend to avoid other foods that promote
cancers. Better studies are needed, and, in fact, one well-designed study that will continue for four years has just been
launched by the Harvard Medical School and will involve 22,000
physicians (see Overview).

In addition to the epidemiological data, however, there are
literally hundreds of papers (many of which are summarized in
Selected Abstracts on Vitamin A and Cancer Biology, National
Cancer Institute, Bethesda, 1979) demonstrating that vitamin
A, primarily of the preformed variety, can suppress the malignant behavior of cultured cells transformed by radiation, chemicals or viruses, can delay the development of transplanted
tumors and can even completely prevent malignancy in animals
exposed to various potent carcinogens. Some of these results, it
should be noted, have been obtained with doses of preformed
vitamin A far too high and too toxic for general, preventive use.
Experiments of the same sort with the far less toxic beta-carotene, meanwhile, appear promising but remain inconclusive
owing to their small number.

Bollag (*Lancet*, Apr. 16, 1983, p. 860) suggests the mode of
action of retinol in regulating the growth and differentiation of
cells and examines a number of new retinoids that may be more

effective and less toxic than preformed vitamin A. Peto and colleagues (*Nature*, 290:201, 1981), meanwhile, suggest that beta-carotene's hypothesized anticancer effects may be due to conversion, in the target cancer tissues, to retinoids, acting like the preformed vitamin A upon mechanisms of cellular differentiation. Or, they speculate, beta-carotene may work in ways unrelated to cell differentiation, by enhancing immune function (see below) or by "quenching singlet oxygen," that is, by putting out one of the primary "fires" of everyday metabolic processes, a fire that almost certainly contributes to aging and degenerative disease, including cancer. As these researchers note, "beta-carotene is the most efficient quencher of singlet oxygen thus far discovered."

2) Speeds healing and fights infections—Population studies have shown that vitamin A deficiency is associated with higher incidence of many human infections (see, for example, *Physiological Reviews*, 60:188, 1980). Numerous animal studies have shown similar associations (*Nutrition and the M.D.*, 8:1, 1982).

Supplementation with vitamin A, in various forms, in doses in excess of nutritional needs, has boosted immunity in some laboratory animals. These boosting effects have included increased antibody activity, faster rejection of skin grafts and accelerated production of various disease-fighting cells (*Journal of Infectious Diseases*, 129:597, 1974; *Immunology*, 23:283, 1974). Increases in cellular immunity were noted in a small study in which lung-cancer patients were given extraordinarily high doses (1.5 million IUs daily) of vitamin A for three weeks (*Oncology*, 34:234, 1977). Doses of preformed vitamin A in that range require constant medical supervision and cannot be tolerated for long periods.

Accelerated wound healing has been observed in animals given supplemental beta-carotene. The acceleration was significant, but these are animals that are deficient in vitamin A to begin with. Diabetics are noted for having slow-healing wounds and for being particularly prone to infections; so are surgical patients. Animal work at Albert Einstein College of Medicine in New York suggests that supplemental vitamin A might benefit these patients, as it did diabetic and other test animals (*Annals of Surgery*, 194:42, 1981). "We believe," these researchers concluded, "that just as supplemental vitamin A improves immune responses of traumatized animals and surgical patients, it will be especially useful in preventing wound infection and promoting wound healing in surgical diabetic patients."

Evidence has existed for several years that very high doses of retinol could markedly reduce the immune-suppressive effects of radiation treatment, cancer chemotherapy and various surgical anesthetics (*Chemotherapy*, 8:287, 1976; *Surgery, Gynecology & Obstetrics*, 149:658, 1979). Again, however, the doses of preformed vitamin A required to achieve these results were too high and too toxic for routine use. Recently, Seifter and associates at Albert Einstein College of Medicine have achieved similar results in cancerous mice, using nontoxic beta-carotene. Supplementation with beta-carotene reportedly permitted increased dosages of chemotherapy and radiation and complete regression of tumors in most of the mice. Some 92 percent of the animals were said to be cancer-free fourteen months after treatment. Human clinical trials are planned, under sponsorship of the National Cancer Institute.

3) Improves vision—There is no dispute over vitamin A's role in helping to *maintain* vision. Vitamin A deficiency produces night blindness. There is no reliable evidence, however, that vitamin A, in any of its forms, will preserve or restore eyesight except in some cases where there is frank vitamin A deficiency to begin with. Most common vision problems are unrelated to vitamin A intake.

4) Fights skin diseases—Extremely high doses of preformed vitamin A have been shown capable of reversing various forms of acne, but only with accompanying vitamin A toxicity and return of acne symptoms after cessation of treatment (*International Journal of Dermatology*, 20:278, 1981). New synthetic analogues of vitamin A, however, are showing remarkable promise in treating a number of serious skin disorders and with far less toxicity (*Lancet*, Apr. 16, 1983, p. 860). Diseases susceptible to treatment by some of these synthetics include some of the most severe forms of acne and psoriasis. These synthetic substances are still largely experimental.

RELATED TO NEGATIVE CLAIMS:

1) Highly toxic—Preformed vitamin A is unquestionably toxic in high doses, although these usually have to be maintained for

long periods before signs of toxicity begin to appear. There is a high degree of variability from one individual to another. Some take 50,000 IUs of vitamin A daily for years without apparent difficulty, while a few may react adversely to a single 20,000-IU capsule. Signs of toxicity include headaches, blurred vision, nausea, hair loss, itchy eyes, aching bones, sores on the skin. These symptoms usually recede quickly when vitamin A is discontinued. Some of the new vitamin A analogues are less toxic. Beta-carotene, which is exciting so much interest in current research, shows little if any sign of toxicity (D. S. McLaren, in T. B. Fitzpatrick et al., eds., *Dermatology in General Medicine*, 2nd ed., McGraw-Hill, New York, 1979).

2) May cause birth defects if taken during pregnancy—Preformed vitamin A has been linked to birth defects in various animals. In humans, a few cases of defects linked to daily ingestion of 40,000 IUs (or more) have been reported (*CRC Critical Reviews in Toxicology*, 9:351, 1979). There is no evidence that beta-carotene, at any dose level, produces birth defects. Pregnant women, however, should not take any drug, vitamin, mineral or food supplement without first consulting their physicians.

3) May cause bone disease among those with chronic kidney failure—A recent study (*British Medical Journal*, 282:1999, 1981) indicates that kidney patients who are undergoing dialysis may be at special risk of suffering one particular form of vitamin A toxicity—a bone disease that results from increased resorption of bone leading to high levels of calcium in the blood. This hypercalcemia, associated with a high intake of preformed vitamin A, is relatively rare in normal individuals (*Western Journal of Medicine*, 137:429, 1982). The higher-than-expected frequency of bone fractures in *polar bears* is related to their high dietary intake of preformed vitamin A. Patients with chronic kidney failure should consult with their physicians before taking vitamin A.

IV. Recommendations

A) SUGGESTED INTAKE: The U.S. Recommended Daily Allowance for vitamin A is 5,000 IUs. Some "megavitamin" advocates have recommended taking up to 50,000 IUs daily—a dose that definitely could be hazardous in many cases. The RDA 5,000, on the other hand, may be insufficient for many people, particularly those who smoke, those who live on junk foods or otherwise have poor nutrition, those who are hospitalized, those who are recovering from surgery, those who are diabetic, those who are fighting infections, those who are exposed to high levels of toxic chemicals and pollutants. The RDA is based on the assumption that vitamin A will be derived in whole or part from preformed vitamin A, the potential toxicity of which, in high doses, is established. Even where preformed vitamin A is concerned, however, there is virtually no evidence that daily supplementation with *up to* 15,000 IUs will pose any real risk, even in children.

With the recent advent of inexpensive and readily available beta-carotene supplements, and with the accumulation of evidence suggesting that this vitamin A precursor can confer many of the same and perhaps even additional benefits, there is *no reason to take preformed vitamin A supplements at all*, except under certain doctor-prescribed circumstances. Instead, you should eat at least some foods rich in vitamin A on a daily basis (for example, one average-sized carrot gives you a full 5,000 IUs of beta-carotene) and, as a potential preventive against some of the diseases discussed above, take a daily supplement of 15,000 to 25,000 IUs of beta-carotene. This amount can safely be used by children as well as adults. Beta-carotene in these quantities is safe for pregnant women too, but, as noted above, all pregnant women should consult with their physicians about any drugs, vitamins, minerals or other food supplements they are considering. Pregnant women should definitely avoid taking more than 5,000 IUs of *preformed* vitamin A daily during pregnancy.

B) SOURCE/FORM: Fish-liver oil, meats and animal products are the richest sources of preformed vitamin A. Half a pound of calf's liver contains almost 75,000 IUs of preformed vitamin A. Carrots, sweet potatoes, broccoli, spinach, collards, turnip greens, kale, cantaloupe, winter squash, mustard greens, beet greens, papayas, apricots, watermelons, tomatoes and lettuce are among the foods rich in beta-carotene. A single sweet potato contains nearly 10,000 IUs of beta-carotene. As for supplements, there are numerous beta-carotene preparations on the market today. Most of these appear to be of about equal value. Compare prices.

C) TAKE WITH: Try to incorporate beta-carotene into a well-balanced vitamin mineral "insurance" formula. Be aware that high intake of vitamin E (apparently in amounts greater than 600 IUs daily) has been shown to interfere with beta-carotene absorption and utilization. (See Part Three for more specific recommendations.)

D) CAUTIONARY NOTE: Discontinue taking vitamin A, in any form, if signs of toxicity arise, such as persistent headaches, blurred vision, nausea, hair loss, aching bones, skin lesions. Toxicity is *highly* unlikely with beta-carotene supplementation. If you are taking preformed vitamin A (retinol), limit the dosage to 15,000 IUs daily. Discontinue taking *preformed* vitamin A or cut back to no more than 5,000 IUs daily if you are a pregnant woman or a woman using the birth-control pill. The Pill has been shown to increase blood levels of retinol independent of supplementation. Beta-carotene, however, *has not* been shown to have an adverse interaction with the birth-control pill. Also, as noted above, do not take more than 600 IUs of vitamin E daily with the recommended beta-carotene. Vitamin E, in high doses, has been shown to interfere with beta-carotene absorption.

Vitamin B₃ (Niacin)

I. Overview

Niacin is one of those nutrients that, though not household words, have achieved almost cult status in the supplement underground. For decades, some researchers have claimed that niacin can prevent or even cure schizophrenia. More recently, niacin advocates have claimed that the nutrient can cleanse the body of all manner of toxins, pollutants and even many narcotic drugs. Some Vietnam veterans have credited niacin with purging them of "Agent Orange." Recently, the Church of Scientology has reportedly advocated using niacin in combination with saunas to rid the body of various of the pollutants encountered in everyday life. Two authors report using niacin just before sexual relations "to enhance the natural sex flush." More conventional niacin researchers have also found something to cheer about, reporting beneficial effects in heart and circulatory disorders.

The word "niacin" is commonly used to refer to the two forms of vitamin B₃: nicotinic acid and nicotinamide. In a stricter sense, however, niacin refers to nicotinic acid, while niacinamide refers to nicotinamide. (See Recommendations for further details.)

II. Claims

POSITIVE:
1) Helps prevent or reverse cardiovascular diseases; 2) protects against pollutants and toxins; 3) prevents or cures schizophrenia and some other mental disorders; 4) may be of benefit in diabetes; 5) relieves migraine headaches; 6) alleviates arthritis; 7) stimulates the sex drive.

NEGATIVE:
1) Toxic in high doses.

III. Evidence

RELATED TO POSITIVE CLAIMS:

1) Helps prevent or reverse cardiovascular diseases—Beginning in the 1950s, researchers reported that nicotinic acid could lower blood levels of cholesterol and triglycerides, both of which have been implicated in the fatty deposits that narrow the arteries. Favorable results have been reported with doses as low as 2 grams per day. The 1975 Coronary Drug Project Research Group, in a major study (*Journal of the American Medical Association*, 231:360, 1975), found that nicotinic acid measurably reduced cholesterol levels and reduced the recurrence rate for heart attacks among those treated with the substance by 29 percent. Side effects were noted, however, including an increased rate of cardiac arrhythmias (abnormal heartbeat).

Other studies have confirmed the cholesterol- and triglyceride-lowering capabilities of niacin. One five-year follow-up study found reduced illness and death among nicotinic-acid-treated patients suffering from heart disease, as compared with those who did not receive nicotinic acid (*Atherosclerosis*, 38:129, 1980). Another study, involving individuals who were genetically predisposed to high blood levels of cholesterol, has provided preliminary evidence that niacin may be capable of *reversing* atherosclerosis (*New England Journal of Medicine*, 304:251, 1981). Grundy and co-workers, in another recent study (*Journal of Lipid Research*, 22:24, 1981), have reported a niacin-induced cholesterol reduction of 22 percent and a reduction of triglycerides of 52 percent, concluding, "To our knowledge, no other single agent has such potential for lowering both cholesterol and triglycerides."

2) Protects against pollutants and toxins—These claims, though widespread, remain almost entirely anecdotal, and the mechanisms by which niacin is alleged to inactivate and expel these toxins have not been convincingly elucidated. Some claim niacin can vanquish "bad trips" induced by LSD and other "recreational" drugs. Narconon, a Los Angeles drug-rehabilitation program, has reportedly (*Omni*, Feb. 1983, p. 38) used niacin "to detoxify thousands of drug addicts since 1978." It was in that program that two Vietnam veterans claimed to have been cleansed of residues from the toxic defoliant "Agent Orange." According to *Omni*, the Los Angeles-based Foundation for Advancement in Science and Education did a follow-up study on 103 persons who were treated with a regimen that combined niacin, saunas and exercise and found (not surprisingly) reduced cholesterol levels. They also reported reduced blood pressure. More intensive tests on 7 of the study subjects reportedly showed reduced levels of various, previously noted, toxins, including PCBs and such pesticides as heptachlor and dieldrin.

The niacin/sauna/exercise "Purification Program" was, *Omni* reported, apparently named and initiated by the Church of Scientology. The only explanation given for its claimed efficacy is that niacin supposedly frees up toxic substances that are stored in fatty tissues; prolonged saunas and long-distance running then expel the toxins in the ensuing perspiration.

These reports are interesting, even intriguing, but they will require scientific, well-controlled confirmation before niacin can be said to have any real role as a useful detoxifier.

3) Prevents or cures schizophrenia and some other mental disorders—The most striking effect of severe niacin deficiency is the disease pellagra, which is characterized by dementia, diarrhea, depression and skin problems. Pellagra was the first form of "mental illness" to be directly linked to a physical cause: lack of B vitamins in general and especially lack of niacin. Since then a few researchers have persistently claimed that some forms of schizophrenia can also be treated successfully with niacin. There is, as yet, no adequate substantiation of these claims.

4) May be of benefit in diabetes—This is a relatively new claim. It is based on some work regarding a substance called the glucose tolerance factor, which is thought to potentiate the effect of insulin in glucose metabolism (see section on chromium). Glucose tolerance factor was earlier thought to have nicotinic acid as part of its structure. But at present it is unclear whether nicotinic acid is in fact present in glucose tolerance factor, and there is no evidence that nicotinic acid is of benefit in diabetes.

5) Relieves migraine headaches—Some doctors, and others, report anecdotal success in using niacin to abort migraine headaches when they first begin. Unfortunately, there are no controlled studies to substantiate these claims.

6) Alleviates arthritis—There is no evidence to support this claim.

7) Stimulates the sex drive—Niacin is a vasodilator, which means that it expands the blood vessels, increasing blood flow into certain parts of the body. The so-called "niacin flush" is often experienced by those who take large doses of this nutrient. The flush is something like a protracted blush and is usually confined to the face, neck and shoulders. A few, but only a very few, claim that this flush sometimes pervades the genital region as well, and is thus sexually stimulating or pleasurable. Niacin is not recommended for this purpose. The chances of your finding the flush sexually stimulating are extremely remote. Most people find the niacin flush highly annoying (see below); some find it frightening. Moreover, niacin in high doses is not without potentially serious risks in some individuals (as explained below).

RELATED TO NEGATIVE CLAIMS:

1) Toxic in high doses—Those who take nicotinic acid in large doses—usually 100 milligrams or more—experience what has been called the "niacin flush," a burning, itching, reddening, tingling sensation, usually in the face, neck, arms and upper chest, which may persist for half an hour or even longer, causing some people fright and others discomfort. This effect is due to niacin's ability to dilate the blood vessels. The flush is not considered dangerous, but the sort of doses that produce it (greater than 100 milligrams) can, in a few individuals, produce other unwanted side effects, including nausea, headache, cramps, diarrhea. Even fewer report altered heart rates and temporarily lowered blood pressure, which may produce a feeling of faintness. Persons suffering from cardiac arrhythmia (irregular heartbeat) should consult their physicians before taking niacin. Still larger doses of niacin (in excess of 2 grams daily) have been reported to produce skin discoloration and dryness, decreased glucose tolerance, high uric-acid levels, aggravation of peptic ulcers and even symptoms that resemble some of those that accompany hepatitis. There is some evidence (*New England Journal of Medicine*, 304:251, 1981) that liver toxicity can be avoided, even at these doses, through very gradual increases in dosage, arriving at the 2-gram level only after some months. No one, however, should take these megadoses without medical supervision.

IV. Recommendations

A) SUGGESTED INTAKE: The National Research Council recommends 13 to 18 milligrams of niacin for adults, 6 to 8 milligrams for infants and 9 to 16 milligrams for children one through ten. There are, at present, no data to justify the 500 to 3,000-milligram doses some niacin enthusiasts recommend. Large doses may be useful under certain circumstances, when ordered by and supervised by a physician. Very large doses of niacin have pharmacological effects that require careful monitoring by a doctor. Possible, but not proved, benefit may accrue from taking 50 to 100 milligrams of niacin daily if you are eleven years of age or older. Do not take more than this unless ordered to do so by a physician.

B) SOURCE/FORM: Dietary sources of niacin include lean meats, fish and poultry. Vitamin B₃ as a supplement is available in the form of nicotinic acid or as nicotinamide (niacinamide). Nicotinamide, unlike nicotinic acid, does not cause the so-called "niacin flush."

C) TAKE WITH: It is important to take B vitamins in a well-balanced combination, rather than individually. Get your niacin in a good vitamin/mineral "insurance" formula if possible. (See Part Three for further recommendations.)

D) CAUTIONARY NOTE: Discontinue if any signs of toxicity occur, such as nausea, headaches, cramps, diarrhea, feeling of faintness, accelerated or irregular heartbeat. Toxicity is highly unlikely if intake is limited to the above-recommended dose.

Vitamin B₆

I. Overview

Vitamin B₆, made up of pyridoxine, pyridoxal and pyridoxamine, has, until recently, been a rising star in the super-supplement galaxy. Megavitamin enthusiasts have often proclaimed it the most beneficial of all the B vitamins and some have recommended doses more than 2,000 times greater than the FDA's Recommended Daily Allowance, confidently proclaiming that this water-soluble vitamin poses no risk to human health, even in these massive doses. Such claims were short-circuited in mid-1983 with the report (*New England Journal of Medicine,* 309:445, 1983) that large doses of this vitamin can, with prolonged use, cause serious neurological damage in some individuals, proving once again, that there *can* be "too much of a good thing."

And B₆ definitely is a good thing—*in moderation.* B₆ is required for the proper functioning of more than sixty enzymes and is essential for normal nucleic-acid and protein synthesis. It plays a role in the multiplication of all cells and the production of red blood cells and the cells of the immune system. Through its effects on various minerals and brain neurotransmitters, it impacts on the nervous system. Severe B₆ deficiency can result in anemia, nervous disorders and various skin problems. It has been claimed that women have special need of B_6—while on the Pill, during pregnancy and in order to alleviate some of the symptoms of premenstrual tension. Recently some very preliminary evidence has emerged that suggests a possible anticancer role for B_6.

II. Claims

POSITIVE:
1) Relieves the symptoms of premenstrual tension and cures some forms of infertility; 2) has anticonvulsant effects and protects against nervous disorders; 3) helps control diabetes; 4) protects against metabolic imbalances caused by oral contraceptives; 5) boosts immunity; 6) prevents skin diseases; 7) protects against cancer; 8) inhibits cataract development.

NEGATIVE:
1) Toxic in high doses and may cause serious nerve damage; 2) reduces the therapeutic effect of levodopa, a drug used by sufferers of Parkinson's disease.

III. Evidence

RELATED TO POSITIVE CLAIMS:

1) Relieves the symptoms of premenstrual tension and cures some forms of infertility—It has been claimed for some time that B_6 can relieve various of the discomforts to which women, in particular, fall prey. Various disturbances of estrogen metabolism are claimed to be corrected with supplemental B_6. Premenstrual tension, often characterized by breast tenderness, headaches, weight gain due to water retention, and irritability arising in the week to ten days prior to menstruation, is a significant problem for many women. This syndrome has been attributed to a variety of hormonal processes, some of which are known to be affected by B_6. Abraham and Hargrove (*Infertility*, 3:155, 1980) reported that 21 of 25 women given 500 milligrams of B_6 daily, in time-release tablets, in a double-blind study enjoyed significant relief from premenstrual symptoms. Treatment continues through three consecutive menstrual cycles. These researchers have also reported (*Infertility*, 2:315, 1980) that women with unexplained infertility experienced "a high concep-

tion rate" after B$_6$ therapy was implemented. These results need corroboration from other investigators.

2) Has anticonvulsant effects and protects against nervous disorders—It is established that B$_6$ deficiency can cause convulsions and degeneration of peripheral nerves. In fact, it was through the administration of high doses of B$_6$ to infants suffering from convulsions that Hunt and co-workers (see P. J. Garry, ed., *Human Nutrition: Clinical and Biochemical Aspects*, American Association for Clinical Chemistry, Washington, D.C., 1981, pp. 219–38) demonstrated in 1954 the first of many inborn vitamin-responsive disorders of metabolism. B$_6$ supplementation dramatically abolishes seizures in most of these infants. A neurotransmitter in the brain thought to inhibit certain types of seizures depends in part for its existence upon adequate supplies of B$_6$. Except in these cases of inborn metabolic disorder, however, there is no evidence to support the claim that B$_6$ is effective against convulsive seizures in general. There is, in fact, some evidence (*Clinical Pediatrics*, 20:208, 1981) directly refuting this claim. Severe lack of B$_6$ may result in nerve disease, but there is no evidence that supplementation with B$_6$, beyond nutritional needs, confers any additional protection against neuropathy. On the contrary (see evidence related to negative claims below), recent evidence suggests that prolonged megadosage with B$_6$ may *cause* nerve damage.

3) Helps control diabetes—There is some evidence that *some* forms of diabetes may be contributed to by B$_6$ deficiencies. (For a brief review of some of the relevant literature, see *Lancet*, Apr. 10, 1976, pp. 788–89.) Adequate levels of B$_6$ are required for the proper metabolism of the amino acid tryptophan. Abnormalities of tryptophan metabolism, which may contribute to glucose intolerance, have been reported in some diabetics, and these abnormalities have been found to be reversible with administration of supplemental B$_6$ (*Journal of Clinical Investigation*, 40:617, 1961; *Lancet*, 1:897, 1973). Dubuc (*Journal of Medicine Bordeaux*, 138:881, 1961) has reported that supplemental B$_6$ can reduce the need for insulin in some diabetics. Other research (*British Medical Journal*, 2:13, 1975) suggests that supplemental B$_6$ can enhance carbohydrate tolerance during pregnancy, when diabetes can pose special risks. There is as yet no proof that B$_6$ is protective against diabetes; there are studies that

fail to show improvement in glucose tolerance in gestational diabetes mellitus (*Obstetrics and Gynecology*, 50:370,1977) and in pyridoxine-deficient men (*American Journal of Clinical Nutrition*, 38:440,1983).

4) Protects against metabolic imbalances caused by oral contraceptives—Women who take oral contraceptives usually exhibit abnormalities of tryptophan metabolism of the sort discussed under diabetes (above). These abnormalities have been at least partially corrected by administration of supplemental B_6, with resulting improvement in carbohydrate (sugar) tolerance (*Contraception*, 6:265, 1972; *Lancet*, Apr. 10, 1976, p. 759). Daily intake of 5 milligrams of B_6 is generally adequate to overcome this abnormality caused by oral contraceptives, making it clear that the megadoses of this vitamin that are often recommended during pregnancy by enthusiasts are not justified (*Nutrition Reviews*, 37:344, 1979).

5) Boosts immunity—Animals and human volunteers subjected to B_6 deficiency have been found to suffer profound depression of both cell-mediated and humoral-mediated immune functions (*American Journal of Clinical Nutrition*, 35: Feb. Supplement 1982, pp. 418–21). In fact, of all the B vitamins, B_6 appears to be the most important for normal functioning of the immune system. Several disease states are characteristically associated with immune-function deficiencies, for example, certain types of cancer and AIDS (acquired immune deficiency syndrome). It would be of interest to determine if supplementary vitamin B_6 is capable of enhancing immune response in any of these diseases. The incidence of vitamin B_6 inadequacy in alcoholic populations may be as high as 20 to 30 percent, and inadequacy of this vitamin may be a significant nutritional problem in the elderly. These are groups that may also be immunocompromised.

6) Prevents skin diseases—Claims that large doses of B_6 can clear up acne and dry, itching skin have been made for some time—but without objective support. B_6 may help clear up some skin problems but only if there is a severe B_6 deficiency to begin with.

7) Protects against cancer—This claim has originated only very recently and not in the popular but rather in the medical litera-

ture. Disorbo and colleagues (*American Society of Clinical Oncology*, 2:232, 1982; *Nutrition and Cancer*, 5:10, 1983) have found that B_6 can inhibit the growth of a number of different types of cancer cells in culture. Mice given B_6 (in the form of pyridoxal) and then injected with melanoma cells, of the sort that appear in a particularly lethal form of skin cancer, exhibited significantly greater resistance to this cancer than did control mice that did not receive pretreatment with B_6. The vitamin-treated mice had more than a twofold reduction in tumor growth compared to the control animals.

Similarly promising results with *human* melanoma cells treated with B_6 in culture prompted Disorbo and group to test the effects of B_6 in a human subject with melanoma. The B_6 was administered in the form of a pyridoxal cream that was applied directly to the malignant nodules, both cutaneous and subcutaneous, four times daily for a two-week period. At the conclusion of this trial "cutaneous papules were no longer visible" and "the subcutaneous nodules were significantly reduced in size (some nodules showing more than 50 percent regression)." All of this must be accounted encouraging, especially in view of the fact that melanoma has heretofore resisted almost all form of treatment. More investigation is urgently needed in order to further assess these exciting but still very preliminary findings.

8) Inhibits cataract development—It has been suggested that a number of B vitamins may help protect the lenses of the eyes from the clouding effects of cataracts. Research remains very preliminary and, though some positive data may turn up, this claim remains unproved.

RELATED TO NEGATIVE CLAIMS:

1) Toxic in high doses and may cause serious nerve damage—A promotional handout that was available in many health-food and vitamin stores in mid-1983 states: "And since any excessive intake of this water-soluble vitamin is excreted within eight hours after ingestion, B_6 is completely safe and no harmful side effects have ever been reported." This same handout sheet was still in wide distribution, as a matter of fact, some time after

Kaplan and co-workers reported (*New England Journal of Medicine*, 309:445, 1983) nerve damage in 7 patients who had been taking 2 grams or more of B_6 daily. Four of the 7 patients had been taking these doses for only two to four months.

The first signs of neurotoxicity in most of these patients were unstable gait and numbness in the feet, followed by numbness and clumsiness in the hands. Extensive evaluations ruled out the presence of other or additional toxic substances. These patients gradually improved when B_6 was withdrawn, though some sensory deficits remained. The commonest reason given for taking these large doses was for relief of premenstrual edema (water retention). It should not go unmentioned that in two cases women began taking large doses of B_6 upon the recommendation of their gynecologists; in a third instance, an "orthomolecular psychiatrist" recommended B_6. Kaplan and colleagues cite several animal studies in which B_6-induced neurotoxicity has also been demonstrated.

The biochemical bases of this toxicity remain unknown, though various hypotheses are being put forward. One of these, suggested in an editorial (*New England Journal of Medicine*, 309:488, 1983) related to the Kaplan paper, is that B_6 may not in itself be the toxic factor but instead that "an impurity in the pharmacologic product" might be. As the editorial explains, "Before a synthetic vitamin can be marketed, preclinical testing must show that at physiologic doses of the product, a possible two percent impurity is not toxic. But at a dosage that is 2,500 times the RDA, the intake of a two percent contaminant far exceeds the amount that has been demonstrated to cause no toxic effect." At this point, no one should assume that B_6 in its pure, unadulterated state is nontoxic in large doses; even if this turns out to be the case, there is no way for the typical consumer to obtain completely unadulterated B_6 in supplement form.

2) Reduces the therapeutic effect of levodopa, a drug used by sufferers of Parkinson's disease—Vitamin B_6 is involved in the metabolism of L-dopa. If L-dopa is given by mouth, as is the case with patients suffering from Parkinson's disease, the L-dopa is inactivated by vitamin B_6 in the intestine and loses its effectiveness. Therefore, patients taking L-dopa should not consume supplementary B_6.

IV. Recommendations

A) SUGGESTED INTAKE: The FDA's Recommended Daily Allowance is 2 milligrams for adults. Health-food stores typically sell B_6 in 50-to-500-milligram tablets. It is easy to see how an unwary consumer might soon be taking potentially highly dangerous doses of this nutrient—four 500-milligram tablets and you're taking 2 grams a day, the same amount that resulted in significant nerve damage in several patients (see preceding discussion of toxicity). There is nothing in the data to even remotely justify dosages of B_6 in excess of 50 milligrams daily. That is an ample dose for adults, including women who are pregnant or on the Pill. Women who seek relief from the symptoms of premenstrual tension should consult their doctors before exceeding 50 milligrams of supplemental B_6 daily.

B) SOURCE/FORM: Dietary sources of B_6 include meats, whole grains and brewer's yeast.

C) TAKE WITH: Get your supplemental B_6 in a well-balanced vitamin/mineral formula. (See Part Three for further recommendations.)

D) CAUTIONARY NOTE: Don't take B_6 with levodopa, the anti-Parkinson's drug. Discontinue B_6 if any signs of toxicity occur, such as numbness in the hands or feet or unsteadiness in walking. Do not exceed 50 milligrams of supplemental B_6 daily.

Vitamin B_{12}

I. Overview

Vitamin B_{12} has, unfortunately, come to be imbued with the odor of "snake oil," so frequently has it been used by unscrupulous individuals, including some doctors, as a general tonic for everything that ails one. Claims have persisted that B_{12} (cobalamin) is a powerful energizer and rejuvenator, that it can pick one up when all else fails, that it improves memory and ability to reason and concentrate, prevents mental deterioration, and, in general, makes one feel younger.

Vitamin B_{12} is essential in the human body but only in very small amounts. It is, among other things, involved in nerve-tissue metabolism. Deficiencies can result in a variety of nervous disorders and in brain damage; they can also produce a form of anemia.

II. Claims

POSITIVE:
1) Energizes and rejuvenates; 2) prevents mental deterioration.

NEGATIVE:
1) Toxic and a waste of money.

III. Evidence

RELATED TO POSITIVE CLAIMS:

1) Energizes and rejuvenates—There is no reliable evidence whatever to support this claim except in those individuals who have a vitamin B_{12} deficiency to begin with. Such deficiencies are rare; claims to the contrary have no basis in documented fact. Individuals who are suffering from pernicious anemia often benefit from injections of B_{12}. Healthy persons do not. Some individuals who are on a strict vegetarian diet (no eggs, fish, poultry, dairy products or meats) may have a low intake of vitamin B_{12} and a high intake of folic acid, a combination that can conceal a B_{12} deficiency. Such individuals should be particularly vigilant with respect to B_{12} symptoms and should supplement their diets with a well-balanced vitamin/mineral preparation.

2) Prevents mental deterioration—This claim is apparently extrapolated from findings (see, for example, *British Medical Journal*, 1:785, 1966) that B_{12} deficiency can cause memory loss, mood changes, slowing of mental processes and, in severe cases, psychoses. There is no evidence at all to suggest that persons without severe B_{12} deficiency (of the sort that would normally also manifest itself in other serious neurological disorders, including weakness in arms and legs, difficulty in walking, paralysis, etc.) will benefit mentally from B_{12} supplementation.

RELATED TO NEGATIVE CLAIMS:

1) Toxic and a waste of money—There is no evidence that vitamin B_{12}, even in large doses, is toxic when taken orally (by which route very little of it is absorbed by the body). Those who receive intravenous injections may develop skin problems that generally clear within one to two weeks. Certainly "high potency" vitamin B_{12} preparations, "rejuvenation programs" that utilize B_{12} and so on are a waste of money. Megadoses of B_{12} are indicated only in those instances where a genuine B_{12} deficiency can be clinically demonstrated.

IV. Recommendations

A) SUGGESTED INTAKE: Against the 500 to 2,000 micrograms (don't confuse the much smaller microgram with milligrams) that some B_{12} enthusiasts have recommended, the U.S. Recommended Daily Allowance is 6 micrograms. There is no evidence that higher doses will harm you, but neither is there any evidence that they will help you. You'll get all you'll need and more in most multivitamin preparations—5 to 50 micrograms are often included. Don't waste your money on higher doses. Five to 50 micrograms daily are adequate for vegetarians as well.

B) SOURCE/FORM: B_{12} is available from a number of dietary sources, including fish, dairy products, organ meats (especially kidney and liver), eggs, beef and pork. It is not recommended as an individual supplement. Instead, obtain additional amounts in a well-balanced mineral/vitamin preparation. (See Part Three for more specific recommendations.)

Pantothenic Acid (Calcium Pantothenate)

I. Overview

Pantothenic acid is part of the vitamin B complex and plays a number of essential metabolic roles in the human body, including some of those related to the production of adrenal-gland hormones and the production of energy. It has become increasingly popular as a nutritional supplement, widely used for its alleged abilities to boost energy, increase athletic performance, alleviate arthritis and retard aging. Deficiencies in humans can result in abdominal distress, vomiting, cramps, burning pain in the heels, fatigue, insomnia. Signs of reduced immunity to some infectious agents have also been noted in pantothenate deficiency.

II. Claims

POSITIVE:
1) Prevents and alleviates arthritis; 2) boosts energy and athletic ability; 3) retards aging.

III. Evidence

RELATED TO POSITIVE CLAIMS:

1) Prevents and alleviates arthritis—The evidence related to this claim is intriguing. Nearly thirty-five years ago, Nelson and co-workers (*Proceedings of the Society for Experimental Biology and Medicine*, 73:31, 1950) noted that young rats acutely deficient in pantothenic acid suffered defects in the growth and development of bone and cartilage, defects that were reversed with pantothenate supplementation. This experimental work suggested a possible therapeutic role for pantothenic acid in the treatment of human bone and joint disorders.

Some years later Barton-Wright and Elliot (*Lancet*, 2:862, 1963) reported that blood levels of pantothenic acid are significantly lower in humans with rheumatoid arthritis than in normal individuals. From that observation they conducted a clinical trial in which 20 patients with rheumatoid arthritis were injected daily with 50 milligrams of calcium pantothenate. Blood levels quickly rose to normal and relief from many rheumatoid symptoms was quickly achieved in most cases. Symptoms gradually returned, however, when pantothenate was discontinued. (Interestingly, still better results were obtained among arthritic patients who were vegetarians. The best results were achieved among the vegetarians who were given a combination of pantothenic acid and royal jelly. See analysis of royal jelly elsewhere in this book for further details.)

With the exception of studies by Annand (*Lancet*, 2:1168, 1963), attributing relief from symptoms of osteoarthritis in a small number of human patients to oral pantothenate supplements, there was no further work on these promising early findings until 1980 when the General Practitioner Research Group conducted a double-blind study (*Practitioner*, 224:208, 1980) that recorded "highly significant effects for oral calcium pantothenate in reducing the duration of morning stiffness, degree of disability, and severity of pain" in patients suffering from rheumatoid arthritis. Control subjects (who received placebos) did *not* obtain relief in any of these particulars. The oral dose used in this study was one tablet of 500 milligrams daily for two days, followed by one tablet twice a day (for a total of 1,000 milligrams daily) for three days, followed by one tablet three times daily (1,500 milligrams daily) for four days, followed by one tablet four times a day (2,000 milligrams, which equals 2 grams daily) thereafter.

Pantothenate was not found to be effective, in this study, against forms of arthritis other than the rheumatoid variety. Clearly, as the Research Group concluded, further trials are justified and needed.

2) Boosts energy and athletic ability—Anecdotal evidence abounds. Scientific evidence is scarce. In an animal study (*Vitamins and Hormones*, 11:133, 1953), rats given large doses of pantothenic acid survived twice as long as unsupplemented rats when forced to remain in cold water. It is possible that large doses of pantothenate do increase resistance to stress, boost energy and thus enhance athletic ability, but these possibilities have not yet been demonstrated.

3) Retards aging—The claim is that megadoses of pantothenate will retard and remove age pigments, "re-energize" old cells and extend life-span. The life-span claims are based upon a single study conducted by Williams (see R. J. Williams, *Nutrition Against Disease*, Pitman, New York, 1971) in which pantothenate-supplemented mice lived 18 to 20 percent longer than unsupplemented control mice. There was nothing wrong with this study, but it does not by itself *prove* that pantothenic acid can make mice, let alone men, live longer. Clearly, however, pantothenate deserves more research.

IV. Recommendations

A) SUGGESTED INTAKE: The FDA's Recommended Daily Allowance is 10 milligrams for adults. In the absence of any data indicative of toxicity, daily doses up to 100 milligrams do not seem unreasonable as part of a preventive regimen for healthy people. Individuals with rheumatoid arthritis should consult their physicians, calling attention to the literature cited above, before taking megadoses. At present there is no justification for the 1,000-milligram and larger doses that are being advocated by some vitamin enthusiasts; nor is there any guarantee that such large doses, taken for prolonged periods, will not produce hitherto unseen signs of toxicity in some individuals. Megadosing on vitamins and other nutrients is a relatively new phenomenon. Some substances (such as vitamin B_6) that were thought to be completely nontoxic are now being shown to have serious toxic effects in very large doses when taken for protracted periods.

B) SOURCE/FORM: Dietary sources include organ meats, eggs and whole-grain cereals. Supplements are widely available.

C) TAKE WITH: Best if incorporated into a well-balanced vitamin/mineral "insurance" formula. (See Part Three for further recommendations.) Do not take B vitamins singly.

D) CAUTIONARY NOTE: At present there is no known toxicity. This does not mean, however, that large doses are safe. Research on this issue has been inadequate.

Vitamin C

I. Overview

No other substance has been as important as vitamin C in alerting the public to the possible benefits of nutritional supplementation. On the other hand, some argue that no other nutrient has led so many people nutritionally astray; the complaint is that the popularity of vitamin C in large doses has produced a "megadose mentality" that encourages the indiscriminate use of numerous nutrients in quantities far in excess of the Recommended Daily Allowances endorsed by the Food and Drug Administration and the National Research Council. In any event, vitamin C has to be accounted a formidable substance, dominating, as it has, the nutritional supermarket for the past dozen years—despite no end of controversies over claims that it cures, prevents or diminishes the severity of nearly everything from cancer to the common cold.

Vitamin C, also known as ascorbic acid, was the subject of the first controlled clinical experiment in recorded medical history. In the 1750s, a British doctor put limes, rich in vitamin C, in the rations of one group of sailors and then compared this group with a second group of sailors who got precisely the same rations except for the limes, which were withheld. The limeless group, after having been at sea a long period, showed the expected tendency to develop scurvy, a disease characterized by wounds that don't heal, gums that bleed, skin that is rough, muscles that waste away. The sailors whose rations included limes, however, did not get the dreaded scurvy. And thus it was that British sailors became known as "limeys," for they regularly thereafter carried limes or other citrus fruits rich in vitamin C with them on long sea voyages.

Closer to our own time, it was recognized that ascorbic acid could be used to promote the healing of wounds and burns, but it wasn't until the 1970s, when Nobel laureate Linus Pauling published his book *Vitamin C and the Common Cold,* that ascorbic acid became the hottest item in the health-food stores. Thanks in large part to Pauling's claims and suggestions, even if "premature" or not fully substantiated as some have complained, ascorbic acid is now being seriously investigated in leading research centers around the world, with results, related in particular to immunity and prevention of cancer, that, though still far from conclusive, are very promising in several particulars.

II. Claims

POSITIVE:
1) Fights cancer; 2) boosts immunity against colds and other infections; 3) combats cardiovascular disease; 4) speeds wound healing; 5) helps maintain good vision; 6) helps overcome male

infertility; 7) counteracts asthma; 8) protects against smoking and various pollutants; 9) prevents diabetes.

NEGATIVE:
1) May cause kidney stones and gout in susceptible individuals; 2) can cause diarrhea and abdominal cramps; 3) can lead to scurvy in those individuals (and their newborn babies) who abruptly discontinue megadose supplementation; 4) interferes with a number of laboratory tests; 5) a waste of money since the body quickly excretes most of the vitamin C obtained through supplements.

III. Evidence

RELATED TO POSITIVE CLAIMS:

1) Fights cancer—A protective role for vitamin C in cancer is inferred in part from population studies showing that those who regularly eat foods high in ascorbic acid are at lower risk of developing various malignancies, especially those of the stomach and esophagus. Some of these studies suggest that the often-noted high rate of stomach cancer in Japan may be due to diets high in carcinogens and low in vitamin C. The relationship between high cancer rates and low ascorbic-acid intake is reported by numerous researchers (see, for example, *Cancer Research*, 35:3452, 1975; *American Journal of Clinical Nutrition*, 34:2478, 1981). Mettlin and co-workers (*Nutrition and Cancer*, 2:143, 1981) have noted an apparent protective effect of vitamin C against esophageal cancer even after "controlling for" alcohol use and smoking, that is, even after taking these additional cancer-contributing factors into account. Similar findings, again after controlling for smoking and alcohol consumption, were found with respect to laryngeal cancer (*American Journal of Epidemiology*, 113:675, 1981).

Wassertheil-Smoller and colleagues have recently reported major new findings suggesting that ascorbic acid may have a potent protective effect against cervical dysplasia, a condition that predisposes women to cancer of the cervix (*American Journal of Epidemiology*, 114:714, 1981; also see *Internal Medicine News*, 16 [No. 10]:49, 1983). Detailed dietary and nutrient analyses of the women studied revealed that those with cervical dysplasia were significantly deficient only in beta-carotene and ascorbic acid. The incidence of cervical dysplasia was seven times greater among women whose daily intake of vitamin C was less than half the RDA of 60 milligrams than among women whose intake exceeded the official RDA. This finding persisted even after controlling for age, sexual activity and some other pertinent variables. Analysis of results further revealed that women whose daily intake of ascorbic acid is below 90 milligrams (which is 150 percent of the RDA) will have a 2.5 times greater risk of developing this precancerous condition than will women whose intake exceeds 90 milligrams daily. It is estimated, on the basis of current U.S. Department of Agriculture data, that 20 to 40 percent of all women in the U.S. have daily ascorbic-acid intakes *less than* 70 milligrams.

Claims that megadoses of vitamin C can prevent or inhibit familial polyposis (precancerous rectal growths) have not been convincingly demonstrated; nor have claims been confirmed that ascorbic acid can lower the risk of colon cancer.

Cameron and Pauling have reported (*Proceedings of the National Academy of Sciences*, 73:3685, 1976) significant extension of survival time among terminal cancer patients given 10 grams of ascorbic acid daily. The control subjects (against whom the vitamin-C-supplemented cancer patients were compared) in this study were "historical," meaning they were drawn from hospital records. In a better-controlled double-blind study (where the researchers did not, until the end, know which patients had received vitamin C and which had received placebos instead of vitamin C), the Cameron/Pauling findings were *not* duplicated (*New England Journal of Medicine*, 301:687, 1979). This follow-up study, however, has been criticized by some because most of the patients involved had received chemotherapy and/or radiation therapy prior to receiving Vitamin C; these treatments may have so compromised their immune systems, it has been argued, that they could not respond to the ascorbic acid. New studies are under way to test the effects of large doses of vitamin C on terminal cancer patients who have not received prior chemotherapy, thus providing a better test of the Cameron/Pauling results.

The population studies suggesting a vitamin C protective effect against certain cancers are given further support by findings that ascorbic acid, through its antioxidant properties, can block the formation of various cancer-causing substances, principally the nitrosamines, within the body. Vitamin C, in fact, is now added to bacon and some other foods to help prevent the formation of nitrosamines even before they enter the human body. Tannenbaum has recently reviewed (*Lancet*, Mar. 19, 1983, p. 629) the extent and sources of human exposure to nitrosamines. Much has been done to remove or inactivate these substances in malt beverages and cured-meat products, but cigarette smoke and other tobacco products remain major sources of exposure. Some cosmetics also contain nitrosamines. Tannenbaum and others have identified drinking water in some locales as the most significant source of exposure. Tannenbaum cites research indicating that high doses of vitamin C may be useful in protecting against nitrosamine formation in the human body. One gram of vitamin C taken daily has been shown to block the formation of some of these substances in the body (*Cancer Research*, 41:3658, 1981.)

Though the experimental data with respect to ascorbic acid's blocking effects on the nitrosamines are extensive and impressive, the data related to vitamin C's ability to directly inhibit other cancer-causing substances are few and inconclusive to date. There is some evidence that ascorbic acid can suppress the growth of human leukemia cells in culture (*Cancer Research*, 40:1062, 1980), though what, if anything, this portends for clinical treatment remains to be demonstrated.

2) Boosts immunity against colds and other infections—The disease-fighting white blood cells have been shown to be partially dependent upon ascorbic acid for normal functioning. It has also been demonstrated that the level of ascorbic acid in these cells is very often diminished during colds and other infections, after surgery, during pregnancy, and when the body is under stress due to exposure to radiation, drugs, alcohol and cigarette smoking. Leukocyte levels of vitamin C have been shown to decline with age. The assumption has therefore been made that high doses of vitamin C can fight infection and, more important, prevent it. Pauling analyzed (*Medical Tribune*, Mar. 24, 1976, p. 18) a dozen clinical investigations of vitamin C's effects on the common cold and reported a 37 percent average decrease in the *length* of colds treated with ascorbic acid. Numerous other studies have yielded conflicting results. Only a very few have claimed that vitamin C can reduce the *incidence* of colds. Several studies, however, have agreed that ascorbic-

acid supplementation (often in 1-gram daily quantities) can reduce the severity of symptoms and the duration of colds. (See, for example, *British Journal of Preventive and Social Medicine*, 30:193, 1976.) Another study (*American Journal of Clinical Nutrition*, 32:1686, 1979) found that an 80-milligram dose of vitamin C daily is as effective as a 1-gram dose daily in reducing the symptoms and duration of colds.

Some further support is given to the claim that vitamin C may have at least mild antiviral effects by findings that high doses of it can boost the production and activity of interferon, a virus-fighting substance produced by the body (*Infection and Immunity*, 10:409, 1974; *Acta Pathologica et Microbiologica Scandinavica Section B*, 84:280, 1976). Claims that vitamin C can help in the treatment of herpes are given preliminary support by a double-blind study (*Oral Surgery*, 45:56, 1978) in which patients suffering from recurrent oral herpes enjoyed a 50 percent reduction in healing time, as compared with controls, when given 600 milligrams of ascorbic acid daily, beginning when symptoms first appeared. This study needs follow-up, and, for now, we do not know if vitamin C can decrease the *recurrence* of herpes. Claims that ascorbic acid can inhibit or prevent hepatitis have not been substantiated.

There is increasing evidence that vitamin C plays an important role in various immune functions. Stimulation of neutrophils (white blood cells that are the chief defenders against foreign bodies) has been demonstrated in young adults receiving 2 to 3 grams of vitamin C daily (*American Journal of Clinical Nutrition*, 33:71, 1981). Regulation of the foreign-body killing mechanism of neutrophils may, in fact, be the most important role that vitamin C plays in the immune system. There is evidence that ascorbic acid favorably affects the mobility of the neutrophil (*American Journal of Clinical Nutrition*, 35:423, 1982). It is conceivable that the effect that vitamin C has on reducing the severity of symptoms of colds has little to do with antiviral activity but may, instead, have to do with an enhancement of the neutrophil's activity against the bacteria that often follow viral infection.

Recently, researchers at the University of Texas have found that in experiments with monkeys, large doses of Vitamin C (far exceeding nutritional requirements) have been effective in preventing gum disease even when bacterial strains known to be destructive to gums are injected directly into the animals' mouths (*American Health*, Sept./Oct. 1983, p. 31).

More research is clearly warranted.

3) Combats cardiovascular disease—Postsurgical patients given 1 gram of ascorbic acid daily, in a double-blind study, developed significantly fewer life-threatening blood clots than did control subjects who did not receive vitamin C (*Lancet*, 2:199, 1973). More recently, Sarji and colleagues (*Thrombosis Research*, 15:639, 1979) showed that vitamin C can inhibit the activity of blood-clotting agents both in vitro (in the test tube) and in vivo (in the human body; in this case in human subjects given 2 grams of vitamin C daily). In other studies (*Atherosclerosis*, 35:181, 1980, and 41:15, 1982), 500 milligrams of intravenous vitamin C given twice daily have also been shown to reduce platelet aggregation (reducing the risk of blood clots).

Humans with coronary-artery disease have been shown to have lower cellular levels of ascorbic acid than do healthy individuals. Guinea pigs with atherosclerosis resembling that which afflicts humans (with similar arterial lesions and elevated serum cholesterol levels) are usually suffering from severe vitamin C deficiency (*Journal of Nutrition*, 99:261, 1969). Vitamin C supplementation restores normal serum cholesterol levels in these animals, which, along with man and the other primates, are the only animals that do not synthesize their own vitamin C and thus must obtain it entirely from diet. Human studies have been few and have yielded mixed results. At this point there is insufficient evidence to support claims that vitamin C can be of significant help in the treatment of cardiovascular disease, though more research is justified on the basis of some of the positive findings noted above.

4) Speeds wound healing—It is well established that vitamin C plays a crucial role in the body's manufacture of collagen, which is the principal protein "glue" that holds connective tissue and bone together. Therefore it may be anticipated that vitamin C is involved in wound healing. There are a few reports in the literature that this is the case. There is also some evidence that megadoses of vitamin C can substantially speed the healing of burns in the cornea of the eyes.

5) Helps maintain good vision—This is a relatively new claim for vitamin C. There are reports that vitamin C may help prevent cataract formation and may be useful in the treatment of glaucoma. There is no substantiation for these claims.

6) Helps overcome male infertility—This is another new claim for vitamin C. Dawson reported at the American Society for Clinical Nutrition in 1983 (*Journal of the American Medical Association*, 249:2747, 1983) that a common form of male infertility, caused by agglutination, or clumping together of sperm cells, making it difficult or impossible for them to swim to the egg, could be reversed by the simple addition of vitamin C supplementation. Ascorbic-acid levels were found to be a quarter to a third below normal in 35 young infertile males studied. Improvement was noted within a few days of beginning supplementation with 1 gram daily of vitamin C. Within a week, blood levels of vitamin C were normal and so were the sperm. More than a dozen of the men's wives were reported pregnant soon after the vitamin C was administered; other pregnancies were expected shortly. Dawson and colleagues have evidence suggesting that vitamin C enhances the body's utilization of various minerals—especially zinc, magnesium, copper and potassium —that are vital to normal sperm functioning. These encouraging findings require follow-up by others.

7) Counteracts asthma—Spannhake et al. recently reviewed (*American Review of Respiratory Disease*, 127:139, 1983) some of the literature related to this claim, noting that negative reports are now being supplanted by more positive reports showing that vitamin C levels in asthmatics are low and that supplementation with vitamin C can reduce to some extent the airway spasms that characterize the disease. Mohsenin and co-workers (*American Review of Respiratory Disease*, 127:143, 1983) have shown that supplementation with 1 gram daily of vitamin C can slightly reduce airway reactivity to noxious stimuli in asthmatics. Increased airway reactivity is the hallmark of asthma. One study indicates that a 500-milligram dose of vitamin C taken an hour and a half prior to vigorous exercise lessens bronchial spasm in some patients. More research is warranted. Asthmatics who want to test the effects of vitamin C, however, are advised to do so only under their physicians' surveillance.

8) Protects against smoking and various pollutants—Numerous studies have documented the lower blood and leukocyte ascorbic-acid levels of smokers (see, for example, *American Journal of Clinical Nutrition*, 23:520, 1970). These levels are diminished by 25 percent in those who smoke fewer than twenty cigarettes per day; they are diminished up to 40 percent in those who smoke more than twenty cigarettes per day. One study (*Annals of the New York Academy of Sciences*, 258:156, 1975) has shown that vitamin C supplementation can restore ascorbic-acid levels to normal in smokers. Vitamin C's role as an antioxidant in the lungs lends support to the idea that ascorbate can afford some measure of protection against various airborne pollutants. Only the foolhardy, however, will conclude that vitamin C supplementation will make smoking "safe." More research is needed.

9) Prevents diabetes—Blood and cell levels of ascorbic acid are subnormal in many diabetics, but vitamin C supplementation did not in one study (*Metabolism*, 30:572, 1981) have any discernible impact on the disease. There is at present no evidence that vitamin C can prevent diabetes, and there is no known role for this vitamin in its treatment.

RELATED TO NEGATIVE CLAIMS:

1) May cause kidney stones and gout in susceptible individuals —Though many doctors still warn those patients of theirs who use vitamin C that this vitamin will lead, as night unto day, to kidney stones, there is nothing in the medical literature to substantiate this claim. A few people are prone to stone formation and gout (mostly for reasons that have nothing to do with vitamin C), and these individuals may, indeed, become even more susceptible if they take large doses of vitamin C. Individuals with histories of gout or stone formation should not use vitamin C supplements without first consulting their physicians.

2) Can cause diarrhea and abdominal cramps—Vitamin C tolerance is highly variable. Some individuals develop diarrhea and cramping on 500 milligrams daily while others tolerate several grams for prolonged periods without difficulty. If problems arise, cut back on intake until symptoms clear.

3) Can lead to scurvy in those individuals (and their newborn babies) who abruptly discontinue megadose supplementation— There have been isolated cases of scurvy arising under these circumstances, i.e., *abrupt* discontinuance of megadose quantities of vitamin C. Large doses apparently condition accelerated metabolism and excretion of vitamin C so that even if normal dietary amounts of the vitamin are available after discontinuing supplementation some hazard of scurvy remains. Unfortunately, the literature does not define the dosage or dosage period that may predispose one to this risk. If you have been taking 500 milligrams or more of vitamin C daily for some time and wish to discontinue supplementation, do so *gradually*, tapering off over a period of several days. Pregnant women who are using large doses of vitamin C should be aware that their unborn babies may develop "rebound scurvy" after birth unless they too are given vitamin C supplementation (*Nutrition Reviews*, 29:260, 1971). Pregnant women should consult their doctors before taking any supplements, especially any megadose supplements.

4) Interferes with a number of laboratory tests—Large doses of vitamin C may make it difficult to determine if there is hidden blood in the feces; they may also interfere with tests to monitor sugar levels in the blood of diabetics. Anytime you have laboratory tests tell your physician what drugs, vitamins, minerals and other supplements you are taking.

5) A waste of money since the body quickly excretes most of the vitamin C obtained through supplements—This oft-heard criticism of vitamin C supplementation is inaccurate and unwarranted. What we know is that about 200 milligrams of vitamin C daily will *maintain* ascorbic tissue saturation in humans (*International Journal for Vitamin and Nutrition Research*, 50:309, 1980). But the argument that supplementation beyond those 200 milligrams is just going to go down the drain, so to speak, is too simplistic and fails to account for many of the recent reports finding significant effects only at higher levels of supplementation. Blockage of carcinogenic nitrosamines (see discussion above), for example, takes place for the most part in the gastrointestinal tract. Vitamin C's activity in this area is not necessarily reflected in or dependent upon tissue stores of vitamin C or amounts being excreted in the urine.

IV. Recommendations

A) SUGGESTED INTAKE: The National Research Council has recommended 60 milligrams of vitamin C daily for adults and children over four years of age. Most nutritional researchers now regard that as too little for optimal health, though few agree with Linus Pauling that the daily dose should be between 2,000 and 9,000 milligrams (2 to 9 grams). Need for ascorbic acid varies considerably from one individual to another. Exposure to infection, tobacco smoke, environmental pollutants, various drugs, surgery, burns, trauma, alcohol and other "stresses" may increase need for vitamin C. So may pregnancy (but consult your doctor first) and advancing age. Though many people tolerate very high doses of ascorbic acid for prolonged periods, the assumption should not be made that these doses are *always* safe. The best available data suggest that adults and children over ten years of age may benefit from a daily intake of 250 milligrams to 1,000 milligrams (1 gram) of vitamin C daily. Children under ten years of age may benefit from 50 milligrams to 100 milligrams daily. Vitamin C will be best utilized by the body if taken in divided doses, preferably with each meal. Since there is some negative evidence regarding doses of 1,500 milligrams daily for periods greater than two months, doses higher than 1,000 milligrams daily are not recommended. This evidence (*American Journal of Clinical Nutrition*, 37:553, 1983) suggests that a high ascorbic acid intake is antagonistic to the copper status of men. However, no adverse effects of the reduced copper status of men were noted in this study.

B) SOURCE/FORM: Fresh fruits and vegetables are the best natural sources of vitamin C. Some of the research cited above indicates that many Americans get quantities of vitamin C in their diets insufficient to significantly protect against various disorders and pollutants. Hence the plethora of vitamin C supplements currently on the market. Many manufacturers hype their individual products as somehow different and better than all others; some declare that their product is "natural" rather than synthetic, that their product is "derived from" rose hips, acerola and other "rich" sources of ascorbic acid. Some vitamin C products come mixed with bioflavonoids (see discussion of these later in this book) and other substances that are supposed to "potentiate" vitamin C. Do not be misled by these claims. There is no meaningful difference between "natural" and "synthetic" vitamin C; nor do bioflavonoids add anything of demonstrated value to vitamin C. (One study—see bioflavonoid analysis— has, in fact, shown that *synthetic* vitamin C is more readily absorbed by the body than *natural* vitamin C both alone and in combination with the bioflavonoid rutin.) Recently, ascorbyl palmitate has been touted as the "best" form of vitamin C. This is a synthetic substance made by combining vitamin C with palmitic acid (a saturated fatty acid derived from fat and used as a food additive). There is no evidence that this is a better form of vitamin C. One of the best ways to get your vitamin C is in the pure granular form. (See Part Three for more specific recommendations.)

C) TAKE WITH: Best if incorporated into a well-balanced vitamin/mineral preparation. (See Part Three for more specific recommendations.)

D) CAUTIONARY NOTE: Avoid taking vitamin C with *inorganic* selenium; take with selenium derived from yeasts (see analysis of selenium later in this book for more details). Do not take with aspirin, as this may increase the bleeding and intestinal irritation associated with aspirin. Discontinue vitamin C if you have a tendency to develop kidney stones or gout. Suspend use temporarily, according to your doctor's instructions, if you are scheduled for glucose tests or "occult blood" tests (hidden blood in feces), as vitamin C intake can interfere with the accuracy of these tests. If you have been taking vitamin C for long periods of time and want to quit taking it, taper off slowly over a period of days. Scurvy has been reported in a few cases where individuals who were taking large doses abruptly discontinued supplementation.

Vitamin E

I. Overview

The discovery of vitamin E dates to the early part of this century. The finding that it plays an important role in the propagation of the rat species gave this nutrient its proper name, tocopherol, which in Greek means "to carry and bear babies." It turns out that vitamin E does not play a similar role in the human species; for a while many scoffed at the idea that this vitamin plays *any* role in human health. Now evidence is being gathered that vitamin E may be essential for the survival of all oxygen-breathing forms of life.

Vitamin E is an important antioxidant, although its precise function in this regard has been difficult to pin down. There is some evidence suggesting that vitamin E, which appears in many forms, the most active of which is called d-alpha-tocopheryl, may have a more fundamental function than that of an antioxidant. There is the possibility that tocopherol, or a substance arising from it within the body, is of pivotal importance in the production of energy.

The first hint of such a role appeared some years ago. Schwarz (*Vitamins and Hormones*, 20:463, 1962) observed a steadily decreasing generation of energy in the mitochondria of cells in rats deficient in vitamin E. Green and co-workers (*Nature*, 190:318, 1961) believed that abnormal or inhibited flow of electrons in the mitochondrial furnaces of the cells choked the energy-making process that appeared to be dependent upon certain substances, including one called coenzyme Q (see analysis of same later in this book). A substance made from vitamin E in animals is very similar in structure to coenzyme Q. (Personal communication, Emil Fürer, 1963.)

This potentially very important discovery has been lost from view for some time. This early work suggests that without vitamin E the "electrical wiring" of the mitochondrial furnaces may not function or not function well. Fortunately, there have been signs lately that vitamin E's precise role in the production of energy may yet be elucidated. Hornsby and Gill (*Journal of Cellular Physiology*, 109:111, 1981, and 112:207, 1982) report that the efficiency of energy production is greatest in those cells adequately supplied with vitamin E, which, they observe, affects the production of coenzyme Q.

When we better understand the roles vitamin E plays in human health we will be closer to knowing how much of this substance we should take in order to ensure maximal health and life-span. The quest for these answers, unfortunately, continues to be impeded by a polarity of opinions. The more hidebound of the nutritional conservatives, relying upon anecdotes and poorly designed studies of the sort they would normally deride, insist that vitamin E is to blame for a galaxy of ills, ranging from nausea and fatigue to vaginal bleeding, blood clots, breast tumors and aggravation of diabetes. At the other extreme, nutritional true believers, showing they can be equally cavalier with the data, ascribe to vitamin E a plethora of miracles, including beautification of the skin, enlargement of the male sex organ, enhancement of athletic prowess and, incidentally, the cure for cancer.

The truth is quite interesting enough, without all the embroidery. Vitamin E is no panacea—and certainly, as we shall see, some people are taking perilously high doses of this substance—but it *is* being employed in medicine for a slowly but steadily expanding range of ailments.

II. Claims

POSITIVE:
1) Protects against cardiovascular disease; 2) protects against air pollution and other toxic substances; 3) prevents cancer; 4) cures baldness and helps skin problems; 5) prevents diseases of the breast; 6) prevents spontaneous abortion; 7) protects against neurological disorders; 8) increases sexual and athletic prowess; 9) boosts the immune system; 10) relieves muscular cramps; 11) extends life-span.

NEGATIVE:
1) Toxic in high doses; 2) may cause bleeding and delay wound healing; 3) may elevate blood pressure; 4) may cause or contribute to dangerous blood clots; 5) may result in serious lipid and hormonal disturbances.

III. Evidence

RELATED TO POSITIVE CLAIMS:

1) Protects against cardiovascular disease—This is the claim most widely made for vitamin E. It was reported in the late 1940s that large doses of vitamin E could alleviate the symptoms of angina pectoris, the intense chest pain caused by insufficient oxygenation of heart muscle. From there the claims expanded to include benefits in a number of other cardiovascular disor-

ders. With one important exception, these claims have *not* been substantiated (for a well-balanced review of the relevant literature see Bieri et al., *New England Journal of Medicine*, May 5, 1983, p. 1063).

The exception relates to a condition called intermittent claudication, which is characterized by pain in the calves of the legs and is caused by narrowing of the leg arteries. Supplementation with vitamin E in doses of 300 to 800 IUs daily for periods of at least three months resulted in clinical improvement in a number of patients with this disease (*Vasa*, 2:280, 1973). The patients who got vitamin E in this study required far fewer amputations than did those who were treated with other substances or with placebos. The vitamin-E-treated patients were better able than the others to walk without pain, and blood flow through the arteries of their legs was significantly improved in most cases, although it sometimes took as many as twenty-five months of supplementation before this improvement was apparent. (For a more recent review of the literature on vitamin E and claudication see L. J. Machlin, ed., *Vitamin E: A Comprehensive Treatise*, Marcel Dekker, New York, 1980, p. 520.)

Claims that vitamin E works to prevent atherosclerosis (narrowing of arteries caused by fatty deposits therein) by lowering cholesterol and various blood lipids have not been substantiated. A recent report (*American Journal of Clinical Pathology*, 79:714, 1983) indicates, in fact, that supplementary vitamin E does *not* alter lipid patterns in normal individuals.

There are several studies, however, showing that vitamin E can help protect against potentially life-threatening blood clots. (See review in *New England Journal of Medicine*, 305:173, 1981.) The nature of this role appears to be quite complex. There is evidence (*Annals of the New York Academy of Sciences*, 393:121, 1982) that vitamin E deficiency is associated with increased aggregation of blood platelets (predisposing to clots). There is also evidence that vitamin E intake can affect two of the prostaglandins (substances made from the essential fatty acids and involved in numerous human biological processes) that have opposite effects on clotting factors. In one study (*Annals of the New York Academy of Sciences*, 393:209, 1982) it was shown that vitamin E's effects on these prostaglandins is evident even in normal individuals. The significance of this remains to be sorted out. Finally, it has also been noted (see Fürer cited in Overview) that, at least in the animals that were studied, vitamin E produces a substance that is similar in structure to vitamin K, which also plays an important role in the clotting of blood. The significance of this link has so far not been investigated.

More research is warranted. Until we have more and better information no one can convincingly claim that supplemental vitamin E will protect *normal* individuals from cardiovascular disease.

2) Protects against air pollution and other toxic substances— There is evidence in some animal and test-tube studies that vitamin E can protect against some environmental toxins. Vitamin E helps block the formation of nitrosamines from nitrates and nitrites, both of which have been used as food preservatives. High dietary intake of these substances has been associated with a high rate of gastric cancer in certain parts of the world. However, only now are well-designed studies being performed to determine if supplemental vitamin E with each meal will result in a decreased incidence of gastric cancer. A role for vitamin E as a protector against various environmental toxins is certainly not out of the question. Only continued research will define that role.

3) Prevents cancer—See discussion of toxic substances above. Clement and Horvath (*American Association of Cancer Research*, 24:96, 1983) have reported that vitamin E alone does not prevent the formation of rat mammary cancers induced by the chemical carcinogen DMBA. They add, however, that it does potentiate the ability of the mineral selenium (see analysis later in this book) to inhibit these tumors. The mechanism by which it does this has not yet been explained. There is some evidence that vitamin E can inhibit a potentially precancerous condition in humans. (See discussion of breast disease below.) Vitamin E is certainly not a cure for cancer. Nor has its possible cancer-preventing capacity yet been substantiated. More research is needed and warranted.

4) Cures baldness and helps skin problems—Vitamin E has no demonstrated effect on hair loss and baldness. Claims of favorable effects on skin remain purely anecdotal. So do claims that vitamin E promotes healing of burns and cuts and minimizes scar tissue.

5) Prevents diseases of the breast—One form of breast disease (fibrocystic) has been shown to be treatable by vitamin E. This disorder, also known as mammary dysplasia, afflicts a significant number of women. The word "dysplasia" connotes abnormal growth of cells. There is concern that in some instances mammary dysplasia may progress to malignancy, although it often does not. Findings that vitamin E may be able to arrest this abnormal development command serious attention. Abrams (*New England Journal of Medicine*, 272:1080, 1965) reported on the beneficial use of vitamin E in this disease. There has been more recent confirmation (*Lipids*, 16:223, 1981). London and co-workers (*Cancer Research*, 41:3811, 1981) report that 600 milligrams (895 IUs) of vitamin E daily is a safe and effective treatment for this disorder, leading to relief of 70 percent of those treated. These studies have a strong subjective component in that they have relied for signs of "clinical response" upon patient reports of reduced discomfort..Objective regression of the disease has also been observed, however, in 10 of 28 patients in a double-blind study (*Journal of the American Medical Association*, 244:1077, 1980). The amount of vitamin E used in this study was 600 IUs daily. More study is needed to confirm these promising findings.

6) Prevents spontaneous abortion—There is no evidence that this is true in women with other than severe vitamin E deficiencies.

7) Protects against neurological disorders—Muller and co-workers (*Lancet*, Jan. 29, 1983, p. 225) reported that vitamin E plays a crucial role in normal neurological functions in humans, as well as many other animals. Various neurological disorders arise in humans deficient in vitamin E and may, these researchers note, be arrested or reversed via prompt vitamin E treatment. Among those who may exhibit vitamin E deficiencies of the sort that contribute to nerve damage are patients with chronic disorders of fat absorption, chronic liver disease and cystic fibrosis. Other researchers have confirmed these important new findings, and physicians are being advised to be aware of the possibility of vitamin E deficiency in their patients with malabsorption/maldigestion disorders. Increasingly, those at risk of neurological disease will be given vitamin E as a *preventive* measure. These individuals may require very high doses of

supplemental vitamin E, but there is no evidence that persons with *normal* vitamin E levels will gain additional protection through megadose supplementation.

8) Increases sexual and athletic prowess—Claims that vitamin E increases sex drive in both men and women and that it enlarges the male sex organ abound. Unfortunately, there is no evidence to support these claims. Similarly, many have claimed that vitamin E supplements can increase stamina, muscle strength and athletic performance, supposedly by increasing blood flow into the muscles and by improving the "oxygen quality" of each cell of the body. There have, in fact, been a few *uncontrolled* reports attesting to such effects. Again, it is unfortunate that these reports have not been substantiated by more objective, double-blind trials (*British Journal of Nutrition*, 26:265, 1971) like those that failed to find any objective effect of vitamin E on athletic performance. It may turn out (see Overview) that vitamin E plays a hitherto largely unsuspected role of great importance in energy production, in which case those *deficient* in vitamin E might indeed experience a greater sense of energy with supplementation. Frank vitamin E deficiency, however, is rare.

9) Boosts the immune system—Nockels (*Federation Proceedings, Federation of the American Society for Experimental Biology*, 38:2134, 1978) has reported that vitamin E can increase resistance to a number of infectious agents. Others have reported on the possible immune-boosting effects of vitamin E in animals (see, for example, *Scandinavian Journal of Immunology*, 14:565, 1981), but much more work will have to be done before it is established that vitamin E enhances immunity to disease in humans, particularly in view of isolated reports of *suppressed* immunity in some individuals on megadoses of vitamin E (*American Journal of Clinical Nutrition*, 33:606, 1980). There is a possibility that vitamin E does play a role in human immunity. An important mechanism in the destruction of foreign microorganisms in our bodies is the generation of toxic oxygen forms by our phagocytes (cells that literally "eat" foreign invaders). Vitamin E appears to be important in the modulation of this process (*American Journal of Pathology*, 112:287, 1983). Here it may turn out that either too little *or* too much vitamin E is undesirable. More research is needed.

10) Relieves muscular cramps—Remarkable relief from persistent nocturnal leg and foot cramps was reported (*Southern Medical Journal*, 67:1308, 1974) in 82 percent of 125 patients, many of whom obtained nearly complete relief with less than 300 IUs of vitamin E daily. Others have reported similar benefits. Further research is indicated.

11) Extends life-span—Denham Harman (see Chapter One) has found that although giving mice vitamin E lengthens their mean life-span it does not extend maximum life-span. The question of *how much* vitamin E is the correct amount for optimal human health and longevity is a very important one for which there is not yet an answer. The assumption that *more* vitamin E is likely to be better than less is a naïve and dangerous one. Vitamin E has proved time and again just how complex and sometimes unpredictable it is. It may be that we will determine what is optimum for vitamin E only after we have done so for a number of the other major antioxidant nutrients.

RELATED TO NEGATIVE CLAIMS:

1) Toxic in high doses—Many researchers regard vitamin E as nontoxic in doses up to 600 IUs per day. "Reports of adverse symptoms from large doses of the vitamin," write Bieri and co-workers (cited above), "abound in the literature and are largely subjective and based on limited observations. The most commonly recurring complaint is that of gastrointestinal disturbance (nausea, flatulence or diarrhea) of a transient nature." There are few reliable data, in other words, indicating toxicity of vitamin E even in doses exceeding 600 IUs daily. But since there is no "indication" for such doses in normal individuals, supplementation exceeding 600 IUs daily is strongly advised against, particularly in view of anecdotal adverse effects (see below).

2) May cause bleeding and delay wound healing—Persons who are taking anticoagulation drugs should be followed closely by their physicians and especially when they take vitamin E supplements. This applies as well to persons who have reduced coagulation factors. These include those who have vitamin K deficiencies. Even moderate coagulation-factor deficiency may

predispose one to potentially dangerous bleeding if vitamin E is taken in doses greater than 400 IUs daily (*Nutrition and the M.D.*, Mar. 1982, p. 1). Vitamin E has not been found, however, to interfere with coagulation factors in *normal* individuals (*American Journal of Clinical Nutrition*, 34:1701, 1981). As for delayed wound healing, this has been noted in a study with animals (*Annals of Surgery*, 175:235, 1972) and was attributed to an inhibitory effect of vitamin E on the synthesis of collagen, the protein that helps bind tissue together. Delayed wound healing has been reported anecdotally in humans. There is no evidence that this presents a problem for normal individuals.

3) May elevate blood pressure—Again, this adverse effect has not been reliably observed in normal individuals. It has been reported anecdotally in persons with preexisting hypertension or predisposition to hypertension. Vitamin E has also been reported to be dangerous in high doses in persons suffering from rheumatic heart disease. Some who advocate megadoses of vitamin E caution users to begin with small doses and gradually increase them in order to avoid hypertension. Hypertensives are advised to consult their physicians before taking vitamin E supplements.

4) May cause or contribute to dangerous blood clots—Roberts (*Journal of the American Medical Association*, July 10, 1981, p. 129) has reported this anecdotally, noting that he often encounters patients who report daily intake of vitamin E in the range of 800 to 1,200 IUs. Though these and some of the other adverse effects reported by Roberts have not been observed by most other researchers, it would be unwise to conclude that doses above 600 or 800 IUs of vitamin E daily are entirely safe. The popularity of doses in that range is of relatively recent origin, and study of long-range effects of these doses has, necessarily, only now begun. It is possible that while certain smaller doses of vitamin E may have beneficial effects in specific disorders, some larger doses may have adverse effects in those *same* disorders.

5) May result in serious lipid and hormonal disturbances— Again, this is the contention of Roberts (cited above), based on uncontrolled observations. A recent, better documented report (*American Journal of Clinical Pathology*, 79:714, 1983) indicates

that supplementary vitamin E does *not* alter lipid patterns in *normal* adults. It is possible, but unproved, that the high doses of vitamin E of the sort associated with adverse side effects by Roberts—and also by London (*Journal of the American Medical Association*, 244:1077, 1980)—do pose perils in this regard. More research is needed. At present, however, adverse side effects have not been reported when daily doses of vitamin E do not exceed 600 IUs.

IV. Recommendations

A) SUGGESTED INTAKE: The National Research Council recommends 4 to 5 IUs of vitamin E daily for infants, 7 to 12 IUs for children and adolescents, 15 IUs for adult males and 12 IUs for adult females (increasing to 15 during pregnancy and lactation). Some vitamin E enthusiasts, on the other hand, have recommended dosages of up to 3,000 IUs daily. Many people are now taking 600 to 1,200 IUs daily. Prolonged ingestion of these quantities of vitamin E may lead to adverse effects. London (cited above) elucidated one of vitamin E's most beneficial effects (in cystic breast disease) yet cautioned against its indiscriminate use: "Right now you can go to the drugstore and buy thousands of grams of vitamin E and take as much as you want, not knowing that it may affect you profoundly. It may change your lipids; it may, and probably will, alter some of your steroid hormones. . . . Vitamin E is not a benign vitamin that you can take like vitamin C if you think you're getting a cold. It is—and we need to stress this—a pharmacologic agent."

There is evidence sufficient to suggest that vitamin E may play an important role in helping to prevent the development of several degenerative processes associated with aging. Supplementation, however, should not exceed 600 IUs daily—for adults. Children between the ages of one and ten should not take more than 200 IUs daily. Infants should not be given more than 50 IUs daily.

B) SOURCE/FORM: Most of us apparently get about 15 IUs of vitamin E in our daily diets, from such sources as whole-grain cereals, eggs, vegetable oils, enriched flour, leafy greens and many other vegetables. Real deficiencies are rare. If you buy vitamin E supplements you will note that some manufacturers stress the "natural" origins of their products. In fact, however, there is no evidence that natural vitamin E is any better or more active than synthetic versions. Acceptable supplementary forms of vitamin E include d-alpha-tocopheryl acetate, d-alpha-tocopheryl succinate, dl-alpha-tocopheryl acetate and dl-alpha-tocopheryl succinate.

C) TAKE WITH: Best if incorporated into a well-balanced vitamin/mineral preparation. (See Part Three for further recommendations.) Because of widely reported synergistic effects, a daily 100- to 200-microgram dose of *organic* selenium should be accompanied in adults by 100 to 400 IUs of vitamin E daily. Children under seven should not take more than 100 micrograms of selenium with their vitamin E. Infants should not take more than 50 micrograms of selenium daily.

D) CAUTIONARY NOTE: Don't take vitamin E at the same time that you take inorganic iron or the contraceptive pill, if possible, both of which may interfere with vitamin E activity. Take vitamin E several hours before or after you take the birth-control pill or iron supplements. This should not pose any problem as far as the Pill is concerned, but iron may be troublesome since you are likely to get it in a multivitamin/mineral preparation that also contains vitamin E. Fortunately, most forms of iron used in these preparations, such as ferrous fumarate, are thought to be compatible with vitamin E. If you take extra iron, however, that is, iron beyond that which you get in your multivitamin/mineral formulation, you'll derive the most benefit if you take this separately and, if at all possible, on an empty stomach. (See discussion of iron for more details.) Don't take vitamin E if you are on anticoagulant drugs, such as warfarin, or if you have a known vitamin K deficiency (which results in diminished blood-clotting ability) unless your physician approves and carefully monitors your condition. Discontinue vitamin E supplementation if any signs of toxicity occur, such as fatigue, nausea, muscle weakness, stomach upset, skin disorders. Also discontinue if cuts or burns take unusually long to heal or if you experience unexplained bleeding. If you are diagnosed as having blood clots of any kind, alert your doctor to the fact that you are taking vitamin E and do not continue without his permission.

five

MINERALS

Carbohydrates, proteins, lipids (fats, fatty acids, cholesterol) and vitamins are all organic substances. What this means is that they are all compounds of the chemical element carbon. We require, in addition to these nutrients, certain chemical elements in their *inorganic* forms, i.e., *not* bound to carbon. These chemical elements in their nonorganic forms are classified as the dietary minerals. These nutrients participate in a multitude of biochemical and physiological processes necessary for the maintenance of health.

These substances are often grouped in two categories, those that are required in our diets in amounts greater than 100 milligrams per day and those that are required in amounts much less than 100 milligrams daily. The term "mineral" is applied to the former group, while "trace element" is applied to the latter.

Minerals include compounds of the elements calcium, magnesium, phosphorous, sodium, potassium, sulfur and chlorine. Trace elements that are required for human health are iron, iodine, copper, manganese, zinc, molybdenum, selenium and chromium. There are trace elements that appear to be important for other warm-blooded animals. These are fluorine, tin, vanadium, silicon, nickel, arsenic, cadmium and lead. Whether these elements play roles in human nutrition remains to be determined.

Mineral-insufficiency and trace-element-insufficiency states are actually more likely to occur than are vitamin-insufficiency states. Those at increased risk of such insufficiencies include people who eat low-calorie diets, the elderly, pregnant women, people on certain drugs (such as diuretics), vegetarians and those living where the soil is deficient in certain minerals. Vitamins are usually present in foods in similar amounts throughout the world, but this is not true of the minerals and trace elements. Because of differing geological conditions, minerals and trace elements may be scarce in the soils of certain regions and rich in those of other regions. The soil of South Dakota, for example, is very rich in selenium, while the soil in certain parts of China and New Zealand is very poor in this element. Thus, you can live in some areas, eat a perfectly "balanced" diet and still develop mineral-/trace-element-deficiency states that can only be averted through dietary change or supplementation.

There is increasing evidence that those whose nutritional status is suboptimal in certain trace elements, such as selenium, for example, may be at greater risk for certain forms of cancer and heart disease. Suboptimal intake can be due to factors other than soil depletion. These factors are as diverse as the effects of acid rain and the overrefining, overprocessing of foods.

Evidence is accumulating from recent studies that mineral/ trace-element supplementation may help prevent various forms of cancer, heart disease and some other degenerative processes. More of these studies need to be done. The impact prudent supplementation may have on medicine may turn out to be enormous.

Finally, for the purists, it is herewith noted that although the trace elements are classified as inorganic nutrients, some of the dietary *delivery forms* of the inorganic elements are structures in which the element is bound to a carbon-containing molecule. This is true of selenium and chromium.

Calcium

I. Overview

The memory of the red dwarf stars that died more than ten billion years ago lingers on in our bones. The calcium that gives our bones their hardness originated in those stars. Calcium is a major mineral, essential for human life. Apart from being a major constituent of bones and teeth, calcium is crucial for nerve conduction, muscle contraction, heartbeat, blood coagulation, the production of energy and maintenance of immune function, among other things. Severe calcium deficiency may lead to abnormal heartbeat, dementia, muscle spasms and convulsions.

Increasing complexity characterizes the evolution of life. The complex functions of human cells require messengers to mediate and coordinate their responses. There is perhaps no more sensitive a regulator of cellular activity than the calcium ion. It is so sensitive that even a slight change in its concentration can cause a biological event, such as a heartbeat, to occur—or not occur. This highly sensitive command mechanism itself requires very fine regulation, for if the concentration of calcium ions in cells exceeds certain levels, even slightly, those cells can be destroyed via the generation of toxic oxygen forms. Magnesium appears to be the prime regulator of calcium flow within cells. It is this delicate collaboration that may well be the major determinant of the rate at which the cellular flame burns.

There are many groups at risk of marginal calcium deficiency. The elderly, in particular, are vulnerable. As we age we have increasing difficulty in absorbing calcium from our intestines. Add to this the fact that as we age we also have a tendency to reduce our dietary intake of calcium. To compensate for this lack, the body begins taking calcium from our bones, thinning them and making them brittle in the process. Postmenopausal women are often deficient in calcium, as are many aging men. Others at special risk include: users of antacids containing aluminum (*Archives of Internal Medicine*, 143:657, 1983), consumers of alcohol (*Biochemical Pharmacology*, 23:2369, 1974), users of cortisone, inactive people, people on low-calorie diets, high-protein diets and high-fiber diets, people who are intolerant of lactose (milk sugar) and pregnant women.

"Eating" our bones for calcium, rather than getting it from our diets, can have devastating clinical consequences. There is evidence that calcium supplementation is beneficial in decreasing the incidence of bone fractures in postmenopausal women and appears to be indicated, along with other factors, for the prevention of postmenopausal osteoporosis; supplementation is likely to be warranted in general for the maintenance of optimal health and longevity. Calcium appears to have a bright and exciting future in preventive medicine.

II. Claims

POSITIVE:
1) Beneficial in prevention and treatment of osteoporosis ("brittle bones"); 2) natural tranquilizer; 3) useful in the treatment of high blood pressure and other cardiovascular disorders; 4) helps alleviate cramps in the legs; 5) useful in treating and preventing arthritis; 6) helps keep the skin healthy.

NEGATIVE:
1) Produces magnesium deficiency and the premenstrual syndrome in women; 2) causes tissue calcification; 3) forms kidney stones.

III. Evidence

RELATED TO POSITIVE CLAIMS:

1) Beneficial in prevention and treatment of osteoporosis—Bones are not the chemically inert things that many imagine them to be. They are in a constant state of metabolic activity, continually dissolving and re-forming. But as we age there is a decrease in bone formation and an increase in bone resorption. Osteoporosis is the most common metabolic disease of bone; it is characterized by diminished bone mass and the tendency to fracture. Some 25 to 50 percent of all women over age sixty-five are said to be afflicted by it. It is now known that the dietary intake of calcium, as well as absorption of calcium from the intestines, decreases with age and that postmenopausal women in particular require more than the RDA (Recommended Di-

etary Allowance) of this mineral (*Journal of Laboratory and Clinical Medicine*, 92:953, 1978). Calcium supplementation can significantly decrease the incidence of fractures in postmenopausal women (*New England Journal of Medicine*, 306:446, 1982). There is also preliminary evidence showing that calcium supplementation is beneficial in the *prevention* of postmenopausal osteoporosis.

2) Natural tranquilizer—Reports that calcium supplements (or a glass of milk) are good for sleep or to calm the nerves persist but remain anecdotal.

3) Useful in the treatment of high blood pressure and other cardiovascular disorders—Low calcium intake has been linked to high blood pressure. McCarron and co-workers (*Science*, 217:269, 1982) reported that a group of patients with hypertension consumed significantly less calcium than a matched group of subjects with normal blood pressure. Following up on this Oregon study, Ackley and colleagues (*American Journal of Clinical Nutrition*, 38:457, 1983) reached a similar conclusion after studying a California community. Belizan et al. (*Journal of the American Medical Association*, 249:1161, 1983) report that calcium supplements lowered the blood pressure of healthy subjects. Placebos had no such effect in this group. Until more definitive studies are conducted to determine the effects of calcium on individuals with hypertension this claim cannot yet be substantiated. Such studies are now in progress (see *Medical World News*, Aug. 27, 1984, p. 38). A protective role is presently *suggested*.

There is no *present* evidence that calcium supplementation is useful in other forms of cardiovascular disease, although calcium is routinely used during cardiac resuscitation to strengthen the heart muscle. Studies are warranted to determine whether calcium has a role in the prevention and treatment of congestive heart failure.

4) Helps alleviate cramps in the legs—Obstetricians occasionally prescribe extra calcium to pregnant women who complain of leg cramps. Reports of beneficial effects remain purely anecdotal.

5) Useful in treating and preventing arthritis—There is no evidence that supplementary calcium is beneficial in the treatment or prevention of any form of arthritis.

6) Helps keep the skin healthy—There is no support for this claim.

RELATED TO NEGATIVE CLAIMS:

1) Produces magnesium deficiency and the premenstrual syndrome in women—Abraham (*Journal of Applied Nutrition*, 34:69, 1982) is the leading proponent of this claim, arguing that the diet is already too rich in calcium. He believes that because calcium is antagonistic to magnesium a deficiency of the latter can occur, causing the premenstrual syndrome in women. This syndrome is characterized by both physical and sometimes psychological distress prior to the commencement of menstruation. Abraham seeks to support part of his thesis by the finding that osteoporosis (discussed above) is not more common in underdeveloped countries where calcium intake is relatively low. The problems with this argument are as follows: Dietary surveys, as noted above, have documented declining calcium intake in Americans, and particularly in aging American women; there is evidence (cited above) that calcium supplements help prevent fractures in postmenopausal women; and, finally, the fact that there isn't more osteoporosis in underdeveloped nations than has been reported probably has more to do with low protein intake than with anything else. Protein, the consumption of which is high in the U.S. and most developed countries, is known to accelerate the loss of calcium.

There is no evidence that supplementary calcium causes magnesium deficiency or that it is related to the premenstrual syndrome.

2) Causes tissue calcification—There are some who believe that calcification of soft tissue, a phenomenon that is extremely complex and that is part of the wear and tear of the aging process, is related to dietary intake of calcium. The only situation where this may be true is in the context of a frank magnesium deficiency. There is no evidence that dietary calcium is associated with tissue calcification. In fact, this process is common in the elderly consuming *inadequate* calcium.

3) Forms kidney stones—It is true that the majority of kidney stones are formed from calcium. However, the process is still poorly understood, and there is no evidence that stone formation is related to calcium intake (*Lancet*, 2:495, 1983).

IV. Recommendations

A) SUGGESTED INTAKE: The National Research Council (*Recommended Dietary Allowances*, 1980) recommends 800 milligrams daily of calcium. An additional 400 milligrams daily is advised for pregnant and nursing women. Unfortunately, few American women consume even this amount. It now appears, moreover, that the RDA needs revision. On the basis of carefully conducted studies, Heanley and Recker (*Osteoporosis*, University Park Press, Baltimore, 1981) recommend 1,500 milligrams daily in postmenopausal women and 1,000 milligrams (1 gram) daily for premenopausal women. I recommend that men also take 1 gram of calcium daily. The elderly, people consuming low-calorie, high-protein, high-fiber diets, consumers of alcohol and users of aluminum-containing antacids should, in particular, ensure that they get the above-recommended quantities. Supplementation of up to 2,500 milligrams (2.5 grams) daily is safe.

B) SOURCE/FORM: The best natural sources of calcium are milk, cheese, ice cream, yogurt, buttermilk and other dairy products. Other sources include salmon, green leafy vegetables and tofu. One glass of milk contains 300 milligrams of calcium; a slice of Swiss cheese, 270 milligrams. There are several calcium supplements on the market. Bone meal contains absorbable forms of calcium but may be contaminated with lead. Calcium chloride is irritating to the gastrointestinal tract. Calcium carbonate is the most concentrated form as well as the cheapest. It also has the advantage of being an antacid. Calcium glubionate is available as an elixir but is much more expensive. Both calcium carbonate and magnesium carbonate are found in dolomite, a popular food supplement. Although it is important to balance calcium with magnesium—this has always been the big selling point for dolomite—magnesium carbonate is not a very "available" form of magnesium, meaning it is not easily absorbed in this form by the body. Calcium gluconate and calcium lactate are more soluble forms of calcium but are less concentrated in calcium. *Your best bet is calcium carbonate.* Look at the label on the product you are using to see which form is being provided.

C) TAKE WITH: Best incorporated into a well-balanced vitamin/ mineral "insurance" formula. (See Part Three for more specific details and recommendations.) Contrary to popular belief and the claims of many manufacturers, neither zinc nor magnesium interferes with the absorption of calcium.

D) CAUTIONARY NOTE: Patients with unusually high calcium concentrations in their blood should not take calcium supplements. Conditons that cause this include overactive parathyroid gland and cancer. Patients who are taking high doses of vitamin D (not recommended unless prescribed by a physician for a specific medical problem) require medical surveillance when taking calcium supplements. Those who form kidney stones should not take calcium supplements except under a doctor's supervision.

Chromium (And Glucose Tolerance Factor)

I. Overview

It wasn't until the 1950s that chromium's potential importance in diet began to be recognized. Prior to that time chromium was widely regarded as another of the toxic trace metals. In the mid-fifties, Mertz and Schwarz (*Archives of Biochemistry and Biophysics*, 58:504, 1955) reported that glucose intolerance in rats could be corrected by feeding them brewer's yeast. (Glucose intolerance is a decreased ability to remove sugar from the blood for cellular nourishment; it is a characteristic of diabetes.) A painstaking search for the factor in brewer's yeast responsible for this effect finally revealed trivalent chromium in the form of a substance named glucose tolerance factor (GTF). It was theorized that GTF potentiates the activity of insulin, required in sugar metabolism.

Chromium-deficient animals, in addition to having glucose intolerance, suffer from impaired growth, elevated blood cholesterol, fatty deposits in arteries, decreased life-span, and decreased sperm count and fertility. It is now established that chromium is an essential trace element in many animals, including man. It has been reported (*American Journal of Clinical Nutrition*, 21:203, 1968) that chromium supplements can correct impaired glucose tolerance in malnourished children. In another report (*American Journal of Clinical Nutrition*, 30:531, 1977), diabetic symptoms, including glucose intolerance, weight loss and nerve disorders, were reversed in a woman given intravenous chromium. She was a hospitalized patient who had been receiving all of her nutrition intravenously for several years when these diabetic symptoms arose. Insulin itself had no effect.

There is evidence (*American Journal of Clinical Nutrition*, 21:230, 1968) that marginal chromium deficiency is common in the United States, possibly due to high consumption of refined foods. Schroeder (*Journal of Chronic Diseases*, 15:941, 1962) found a dramatic decline in the concentration of chromium in a variety of human tissues with increasing age. At the same time it is known that human aging is associated with a progressive impairment in glucose tolerance, possibly linked to an age-related decrease in tissue sensitivity to insulin (*Journal of Clinical Investigation*, 71:1523, 1581, 1983). Since the supply of insulin itself remains fairly steady as we age, it appears that impaired glucose tolerance itself could be responsible for many of the pathological changes that occur as we age. Diabetics, in many ways, appear to be the victims of an accelerated aging phenomenon associated with such diverse problems as hardening of the arteries and increased susceptibility to infection.

Glucose, like oxygen, has two sides, good and bad. We obviously can't live without it, but in some instances it seems we can't live with it—at least not in good health. It can react with many different types of biological molecules, including hemoglobin, proteins in membranes, even conceivably the nucleic acids DNA and RNA. These reactions damage the tissues. Chromium may help restore some of the body's sensitivity to insulin and thus make better use of glucose.

Factors that appear to contribute to a depletion of body chromium stores include aging, pregnancy, high consumption of refined foods and possibly strenuous exercise. Anderson and co-workers (*Diabetes*, 31:212, 1982) have shown that running significantly increases the urinary excretion of chromium. Although it is still unclear if urinary excretion of chromium is a valid indicator of the nutritional status of chromium, it is a factor that could lead to further chromium deficiency in an individual whose chromium concentrations are already marginal.

Chromium supplementation is expected to assume an important place in preventive medicine. I anticipate much further research with this element and its role in optimal health.

II. Claims

POSITIVE:
1) Useful in the treatment and prevention of diabetes; 2) protective against cardiovascular disease and high blood pressure.

NEGATIVE:
1) Toxic and carcinogenic.

III. Evidence

RELATED TO POSITIVE CLAIMS:

1) Useful in the treatment and prevention of diabetes—There is no direct evidence that chromium prevents diabetes, although there is evidence that it can increase glucose tolerance. The best double-blind, placebo-controlled studies have so far not revealed any favorable role for chromium in the treatment of established diabetes. (See *Metabolism*, 17:439, 1968; *Diabetes Care*, 6:319, 1983.) It will be of interest to see if higher doses of GTF chromium have any effect on glucose metabolism in diabetics.

The most promising studies are those involving elderly subjects. Doisy et al. (*Trace Elements in Human Health and Disease*, 2:79, 1976) showed that impaired glucose tolerance often improved when diet was supplemented with a yeast rich in GTF. Offenbacher and Pi-Sunyer (*Diabetes*, 29:919, 1980) demonstrated a beneficial effect on glucose tolerance in 10 out of 12 elderly subjects given chromium-enriched yeast. No such effect was seen in a group of control patients who did not receive chromium supplementation.

Chromium supplementation may have beneficial effects in younger people, as well, it is suggested by the recent report of Anderson and colleagues (*Metabolism*, 32:894, 1983). They found that supplementation with 200 micrograms daily of inorganic chromium (chromium trichloride) improved glucose tolerance in otherwise healthy, nondiabetic subjects.

Overall, research in this area is promising, but further clinical trials will have to be conducted before it can justifiably be claimed that chromium prevents or improves diabetic conditions.

2) Protective against cardiovascular disease and high blood pressure—The evidence here is contradictory. Some studies have shown favorable effects and others have not. Newman and associates (*Journal of Clinical Chemistry*, 24:541, 1978) have reported that patients with coronary-artery disease have significantly lower serum chromium levels than do healthy individuals. Other investigators (*American Journal of Clinical Nutrition*, 34:2670, 1981) report that supplemental chromium significantly increases the level of high-density lipoproteins (HDLs) in humans. HDLs are considered *protective* against cardiovascular disease. The study was double-blind and placebo-controlled. The dose was 200 micrograms daily of chromium trichloride. The study cited above in *Diabetes Care*, however, did not find any favorable effects on blood cholesterol levels. Further investigation is warranted.

There is no evidence, meanwhile, that chromium is useful in treatment or prevention of high blood pressure.

RELATED TO NEGATIVE CLAIMS:

1) Toxic and carcinogenic—Hexavalent chromium is toxic, but *trivalent* chromium, the dietary form of this essential trace element, has very low toxicity. Long-term exposure to the dangerous hexavalent form may lead to skin problems, perforation of the nasal septum and lung cancer. The trivalent form is not associated with any type of cancer.

IV. Recommendations

A) SUGGESTED INTAKE: The optimal amount of chromium intake is not known. The National Research Council tentatively recommends as a safe and adequate daily allowance for adults 50 to 200 *micrograms* (not milligrams). The chromium intake of a typical Western diet is between 50 and 100 micrograms daily and is probably in most instances closer to the lower figure. Only about 1 to 2 percent of this amount is actually absorbed. There is increasing evidence that marginal chromium deficiency is commonplace. Deficiency is most likely among the aged, pregnant women and persons who indulge in regular, strenuous exercise (such as runners). Healthy young people, as well as the aged, however, have exhibited improved glucose tolerance when taking chromium supplements. I recommend supplementation with 50 to 200 micrograms of chromium daily.

B) SOURCE/FORM: Good food sources of chromium include whole-grain cereals, condiments (black pepper, thyme), meat products and cheeses. Fruits are low in chromium. So are most refined foods. Brewer's yeast is a good source of chromium. Chromium-enriched yeast, which has a higher chromium content than brewer's yeast, is now being produced. GTF chromium (found in brewer's yeast and the specially prepared yeast described above) is far better absorbed by the body than other forms studied. Less than 1 percent of chromium in the form of chromium trichloride is absorbed, whereas 10 to 25 percent of the chromium in the form of GTF is absorbed. About 10 percent of the chromium in brewer's yeast is in the form of GTF. Chromium-rich yeast and inorganic chromium are currently available. I recommend supplementation with chromium-rich yeast.

C) TAKE WITH: Best if taken with a well-balanced vitamin/mineral "insurance" formula. (See Part Three for specific recommendations.)

D) CAUTIONARY NOTE: The chemical structure of GTF is not known, thus, to determine its activity, a biological and not a chemical assay is performed. Specifically, fat cells are used in this procedure. There are some yeast products on the market that claim to have most of the chromium in the form of GTF. If a chemical analysis was used to determine this, the claim is necessarily *invalid*. In short, there are some yeast products on the market that are questionable.

Copper

I. Overview

Growing up in New York City I always marveled at the bronze sculptures decorating many of the older buildings. I was particularly fascinated by the greenish-blue crust enveloping these artifacts, which I learned was caused by the slow combination of the copper with carbon and oxygen, an aging process. Later, when I became a trumpet player, I discovered the beauty that could be made by blowing my breath through a copper tube. The relation between copper and oxygen runs very deeply in human biology.

Copper is an essential trace mineral for humans. It plays a singular role in respiration. The protein hemoglobin carries most of the oxygen in the blood and relies upon copper as well as iron for its synthesis and function. Copper is also involved in the production of collagen, the protein responsible for functional integrity of bone, cartilage, skin and tendon; elastin, the protein that is mainly responsible for the elastic properties of the blood vessels, lungs and skin; the neurotransmitter noradrenalin, a key molecule in the working of the nervous system; and melanin formation (pigment found in the skin and hair). Copper helps protect against the ravages of oxidant damage through the enzyme copper-zinc superoxide dismutase, as well as the protein ceruloplasmin.

Human copper deficiency has been demonstrated. The relatively recent clinical practice of feeding patients through their veins has resulted in dramatic demonstrations of the need for trace elements in human nutrition. Copper deficiency is the second commonest trace-metal deficiency that occurs during intravenous feeding. (Zinc is the commonest.) Symptoms of copper deficiency include an anemia that is responsive to iron, lowered white-blood-cell count and loss of bone density (osteoporosis). Copper deficiency has been noted in patients taking zinc supplements (150 milligrams daily of elemental zinc) for periods greater than a year. (Zinc is antagonistic to copper.) Symptoms in this context are anemia and decrease in high-density lipoproteins, which are known to be protective against coronary heart disease.

On the darker side, copper has been called a "culpable heavy metal" that can cause certain types of schizophrenia and heart disease. Indeed, in a *rare* genetic disorder of copper metabolism called Wilson's disease, excessive copper accumulates in the liver and brain, severely damaging both organs. However, there is no reliable evidence to link excessive copper to any form of schizophrenia or heart disease.

Recent studies have shown a wide variation in dietary copper intake. Many individuals may be consuming suboptimal amounts—not low enough to cause overt deficiency symptoms but possibly low enough to affect life-span. Apart from its role as an antioxidant and *possible* protector against some forms of cancer and heart disease, copper's folk-remedy reputation as an anti-arthritic agent may turn out to have some scientific validity.

II. Claims

POSITIVE:
1) Important antioxidant; 2) anticancer substance; 3) protective against cardiovascular disease; 4) anti-inflammatory and useful against some forms of arthritis; 5) immune booster.

NEGATIVE:
1) Promotes oxidation; 2) causes cancer; 3) contributes to schizophrenia; 4) toxic.

III. Evidence

RELATED TO POSITIVE CLAIMS:

1) Important antioxidant—Refer to Part One for a discussion of antioxidants and their anti-aging effects. There is evidence that supports a fundamental role for copper in the protection against oxidant damage of cells and tissue. A large percentage of copper is bound to the protein ceruloplasmin, named for the heavenly blue color created by the copper. Copper itself regulates the synthesis of this protein, which has several vital func-

tions. It is important for the transport of copper in the blood and is involved in the synthesis of the oxygen-carrying protein hemoglobin. By oxidizing iron, ceruloplasmin inhibits free-radical formation from reduced iron. It is, in fact, the most important blood antioxidant. It prevents peroxidation (rancidity) of polyunsaturated fatty acids and maintains the integrity of cell membranes.

Recently it has been reported (*American Review of Respiratory Disease*, 126:316, 1982) that copper deficiency can produce emphysema (destruction of the elastic recoil properties of the lungs, resulting in diminished oxygen transfer from the air into the blood) in pigs. Copper deficiency may be at the base of this because ceruloplasmin appears to be necessary to maintain a protein (called alpha-one-antitrypsin) that seems to help prevent the sort of lung damage seen in emphysema. Thus, ceruloplasmin could be an important lung defense in people chronically exposed to oxidants (such as cigarette smoke and air pollution).

Finally, ceruloplasmin is one of the "acute-phase reactants." This means that the amount of ceruloplasmin available increases in direct proportion to such pathological "insults" to the body as infection, trauma, vascular insufficiency. Production of oxygen radicals and inflammation attend these insults. Ceruloplasmin acts as something of a fire extinguisher—an emergency antioxidant. Copper-zinc superoxide dismutase is a human enzyme that protects against superoxide-induced cellular damage. It has both antioxidant and anti-inflammatory properties and loses its potency when copper is removed from its structure. (See anti-inflammatory discussion below for further details.)

Probably the most important factor in protecting against free-radical generation and damage is the high degree of structural organization of the cell that has evolved over billions of years. One may expect that in the final reaction of respiration, free-oxygen radicals would be generated. This does not occur as long as the structural integrity of the membrane where the reaction takes place remains intact. Copper is an essential factor in preserving the integrity of this membrane.

2) Anticancer substance—Several reports suggest that copper may protect against cancer. Fare (*British Journal of Cancer*, 18:782, 1964) observed that supplementary copper (copper acetate) in the diets of rats protected them against chemical-caused cancers. Levinson (*Nature*, 227:1023, 1976) noted that several

copper-containing compounds prevented the malignant trans-formation of chick-embryo cells by the cancer-causing (to chicks) Rous sarcoma virus. This is of interest because there is increasing evidence that RNA viruses similar to the Rous sar-coma virus may have some role in human cancers.

There are other studies demonstrating that high levels of cop-per salts added to the diets of animals provided protection against carcinogenesis. Most recently, Kensler and colleagues (*Science*, 221:75, 1983) found that a copper-salicylate derivative inhibited tumor promotion in mice. The speculation is that these compounds protect against cancer by acting as scavengers of free radicals thought to be involved in the promotion of can-cer.

There is no direct evidence of a cancer-protective role for supplemental copper in human nutrition as yet. But in view of the fact that substances such as ceruloplasmin and superoxide dismutase are important protectors against oxidant damage, and that free-radical mechanisms appear important in the promo-tion of cancer, further research on the possible anticarcinogenic role of copper is warranted.

3) Protective against cardiovascular disease—Hooper and co-workers (*Journal of the American Medical Association*, 244:1960, 1980) reported that copper deficiency in young men (produced by taking 160 milligrams daily of zinc, a copper antagonist, for a protracted period) contributed to a significant lowering of the level of high-density lipoprotein (HDL). HDL is believed to be protective against coronary heart disease. Klevay (*American Journal of Clinical Nutrition*, 26:1060, 1973, and 28:764, 1975) demonstrated an increase in cholesterol levels in rats fed diets elevated in zinc and low in copper. He concluded that an im-balance in the zinc-to-copper ratio increases the risk of coronary heart disease by lowering the amount of protective HDL. These significant studies deserve further investigation and indicate that the intake of zinc to copper be carefully balanced at a ratio of about 10:1—milligram to milligram. (See Recommendations later in this discussion of copper.)

4) Anti-inflammatory and useful against some forms of arthritis —The use of copper bracelets in the folk-remedy treatment of arthritis has persisted despite the skepticism of most doctors. It turns out there might be something to it, after all. Walker and

Keats (*Agents and Actions*, 6:454, 1976) found a) that the clinical condition of those suffering from arthritis (mainly osteoarthritis, or degenerative joint disease) who habitually wore the copper bracelets became significantly worse after discontinuing their use; b) the worsening effects were not seen in those subjects who had worn placebo bracelets (made of a different but similar-appearing metal); and c) there was evidence that copper from the bracelets, when dissolved in sweat, could be absorbed through the skin.

A number of studies have shown that victims of rheumatoid arthritis (there are five million such individuals in the U.S. alone) have increased blood levels of both copper and ceruloplasmin (discussed in the Overview). The copper content of the synovial fluid of the joints is also significantly elevated in these individuals. For a while researchers thought these higher levels meant that copper was one of the *causes* of arthritis. Now just the opposite is believed—that copper is a protector and that the higher levels are indicative of the body's rallying copper in an attempt to fight off the disease. Copper seems to play an important role in the body's response to inflammatory disease. Ceruloplasmin, to which copper is bound, is a scavenger of the sort of toxic oxygen radicals that are liberated in various disease processes, such as arthritis.

This possibility—that elevation of copper-related ceruloplasmin is a protective response—has stimulated the development of a number of copper-containing complexes designed to treat rheumatoid arthritis. Sorenson has been the major pioneer in this area. (See *Progress in Medicinal Chemistry*, 15:211, 1978.) Copper complexes of aspirin, tryptophan and even penicillamine have been found to have anti-inflammatory activity in animals.

Some very promising studies using copper superoxide dismutase as an antioxidant and anti-inflammatory agent are being carried out. That superoxide dismutase (SOD) is essential to protect against oxidant and probably also inflammatory damage is established. Taking SOD by mouth, however, does not make sense (although this hasn't stopped food-supplement establishments from selling SOD or people from buying it in large numbers; see analysis of SOD later in this book). SOD is an enzyme that gets digested in the gut and thus in the oral form never reaches the target cells and joints. (See *American Journal of Clinical Nutrition*, 37:5, 1983.) *Injections* of copper-zinc SOD (known as Orgotein) directly into arthritic joints, however, have shown *some* effectiveness in trials of patients with osteoarthritis and rheumatoid arthritis (*Clinics in Rheumatic Disease*, 6:465, 1980; *American Journal of Medicine*, 74:124, 1983).

Michelson and colleagues (*Acta Physiologica Scandinavica*, 492:67, 1980) have packaged bovine copper SOD in liposomes (artificial membranelike structures) and, by injecting these sub-cutaneously, have had some success in the treatment of such serious diseases as systemic lupus erythematosus, Crohn's disease, scleroderma, dermatomyositis and severe radiation-induced necrosis (wasting of tissue). Some of these conditions are similar in some respects to some of the arthritic conditions. (See also *Semaine des Hopitaux*, 59:277, 1983.)

Clearly, extensive clinical trials are needed to further define the potentially important role of copper and copper SOD in these diseases.

5) Immune booster—Data on the role of copper in the immune system are very sparse. In spontaneous and controlled experiments with *Salmonella typhimurium* infection in rats, copper deficiency results in high mortality (*British Journal of Experimental Pathology*, 51:229, 1970). Copper deficiency has also been shown to result in decreased antibody response in mice (*Nutrition Research*, 2:721, 1982; *Science*, 213:559, 1981). Thus, copper does appear to affect the immune system, but its role needs clarification. There is no human work in this area, as yet.

RELATED TO NEGATIVE CLAIMS:

1) Promotes oxidation—Up until now I have been talking about the role of copper tightly bound to substances such as copper-zinc SOD and ceruloplasmin. Copper in this form has antioxidant properties. Copper may, however, exist in a form where it is *not* bound—copper ions. These ions can be powerful generators of oxygen radicals and thus promoters of oxidation. In fact, it has been suggested that the copper contraceptive loop (IUD) kills sperm by its generation of oxygen radicals. The role free copper ions play in generating oxygen radicals is unknown.

2) Causes cancer—Margalioth et al. (*Cancer*, 52:868, 1983) examined copper and zinc levels in malignant and normal tissue and found significantly elevated levels of copper in the cancer

of the large bowel, bladder and female reproductive organs but not in cancer of the breast, kidney and testis. There was no difference in zinc levels between malignant and normal tissue. These researchers hypothesize that copper-ion generation of free radicals may be involved in carcinogenesis.

Elevated copper levels in the blood have been found in many different types of cancer, including Hodgkin's disease, lymphoma, multiple myeloma, leukemia, lung cancer, breast cancer and cancer of the digestive system. It is quite possible, however, that these elevated levels are the consequence and not the cause of the disease process.

Schrauzer and co-workers (*Bioinorganic Chemistry*, 7:35, 1977) correlated per capita intake of copper with cancer mortality rates in twenty-seven countries and found direct associations for leukemia and cancer of the intestine, breast and skin. They proposed that copper is involved in carcinogenesis, not by a direct mechanism but by antagonizing selenium, thereby diminishing selenium's protective effects against cancer. (See analysis of selenium later in this book.)

At present there is no convincing evidence suggesting that dietary copper causes or contributes in any way to any form of cancer.

3) Contributes to schizophrenia—Although several researchers have reported elevated serum copper in some schizophrenic patients, these elevations are most likely nonspecific. There is no evidence of a cause-and-effect relationship. A recent study showed no elevation of copper in the cerebrospinal fluid of a range of schizophrenic patients (*American Journal of Psychiatry*, 140:754, 1983). There is no evidence that copper is the cause of any form of mental disease.

4) Toxic—Although copper is toxic to aquatic species and sheep, it is relatively nontoxic in humans. No adverse effects in humans would be expected from a copper intake of up to 35 milligrams daily for an adult (*WHO Technical Report Series*, No. 462, Geneva, 1971).

IV. Recommendations

A) SUGGESTED INTAKE: The National Research Council lists the estimated safe and adequate daily intake of copper for adults and children eleven years and older as 2 to 3 milligrams; 2 to 2.5 milligrams for children between seven and ten; 1.5 to 2 milligrams for children between four and six; 1 to 1.5 milligrams for children between one and three and .5 to 1 milligram for infants. These amounts appear to be sufficient to prevent copper *deficiency*. The *optimal* copper intake for maximal longevity with minimal disease, however, has not yet been defined. As previously noted, there are studies showing that many people may have much lower intakes than those recommended. This is particularly true of the elderly population. Substances that interfere with copper absorption and utilization include phytates (cereals, vegetables), fiber, zinc, molybdenum, cadmium and vitamin C. A recent report showed that young men taking 500 milligrams of vitamin C three times a day for two months developed decreased serum copper and ceruloplasmin which increased when they stopped taking this vitamin (*American Journal of Clinical Nutrition*, 37:532, 1983).

Copper supplementation is prudent. Since I advocate taking 15 to 30 milligrams of zinc daily, I recommend taking 2 to 3 milligrams of copper daily (adult dose) to maintain the zinc-to-copper ratio of about 10:1 discussed earlier. This puts my recommendation, for all age groups, in the same range as that recommended by the National Research Council. Consult your physician before taking higher doses. If a physician recommends higher amounts of zinc than 30 milligrams daily, adjust the copper intake accordingly. Remember: You want to take ten times as much zinc as copper.

B) SOURCE/FORM: The best natural sources of copper include animal livers, crustaceans, shellfish, nuts, fruits, oysters, kidneys and dried legumes. Cow's milk is poor in copper. There are several copper supplements on the market; they all have similar bioavailability and include copper gluconate and copper sulfate.

C) TAKE WITH: Best incorporated into a well-balanced vitamin/mineral "insurance" formula; see Part Three. Because of the antagonisms reported to exist, I suggest that a daily dose of 2 to 3 milligrams of copper be accompanied by 15 to 30 milligrams of zinc, 200 *micrograms* of selenium and 50 *micrograms* of molybdenum.

D) CAUTIONARY NOTE: Copper supplements should not be used by patients with hepatolenticular degeneration (Wilson's disease).

Iron

I. Overview

> "Gold is for the mistress—silver for the maid—
> Copper for the craftsman, cunning at his trade."
> "Good!" said the Baron, sitting in his hall,
> "But Iron—Cold Iron—is master of them all."
>
> —RUDYARD KIPLING,
> *"Cold Iron"*

> It is with fire that blacksmiths iron subdue
> Unto fair form, the image of their thought.
>
> —MICHELANGELO
> *Sonnet 59*

Iron has journeyed together with copper and oxygen for a very long time. It is thought that some of the earliest proteins formed on this planet some three billion years ago contained iron and that soon afterward copper-containing proteins evolved. Iron and copper appear to have participated very closely together in the evolution of aerobic life.

There is a remarkable parallel in the history of human civilization. Iron and copper are the backbone of civilized life. One of the greatest achievements in human history was the ability to work copper by heating it with fire and to create from this marriage the very tools, vessels, utensils and ornaments that have themselves catalyzed the cultural evolution of man. This period became known as the Bronze Age and was succeeded by the Iron Age when man learned how to work iron to produce steel.

The alchemists were concerned with another metal, gold. These medieval philosophers-scientists-magicians sought to change base metals into gold. They saw in this a way of converting the corruptible to the incorruptible, a means of extracting the permanent, the eternal, from mutable, everyday life. But, in fact, gold is worthless compared with iron, for nature, the greatest alchemist of them all, has transformed iron into life.

Respiration is the process of burning foodstuffs (carbohydrates, fats, proteins) to produce biological energy without which life could not be sustained. Iron is involved in the entire process of respiration. It is the backbone of the energy-producing process. Hemoglobin is the protein that carries most of the oxygen in the red blood cells; its function and synthesis depend profoundly on iron. The basic reaction that produces energy in the metabolic furnaces of the cells—the mitochondria—is the combination of oxygen with hydrogen to form water. This reaction occurs by means of a flow of electrons, derived from the oxidation of foodstuffs, across electron-carrier proteins called cytochromes and via the final combination of these electrons with oxygen, catalyzed by an enzyme called cytochrome oxidase, to produce water. The cytochromes and cytochrome oxidase do not work without iron, which, in turn, depends in some particulars upon a collaboration with copper.

Apart from its fundamental role in biological energy production, iron is involved in the production of carnitine (see analysis of carnitine later in this book), a small molecule that is necessary for the oxidation of fatty acids. Iron plays roles in the production of collagen and elastin, two major components necessary for the integrity of connective tissue, in the maintenance of the immune system, in the production and regulation of several brain neurotransmitters, and in the protection against oxidant damage.

That iron is a trace mineral essential for human health is firmly established. The condition most commonly associated with iron deficiency—iron-deficiency anemia—was described by Egyptian physicians at the very beginning of the Iron Age, 1500 B.C. Of course they did not know that they were diagnosing an iron-deficiency anemia, but the symptoms they described, such as pallor and difficulty in breathing, were almost certainly due to this disorder. Iron was identified as having an important role in human health in the middle of the seventeenth century when Thomas Sydenham recommended iron supplementation as a specific remedy for chlorosis, or green sickness (iron-deficiency anemia). Iron deficiency is frequently seen in infants, adolescents and pregnant women. Iron supplementation is particularly recommended for these groups. It should be noted that iron deficiency can also occur *without* anemia, producing such symptoms as fatigue, behavioral problems (decreased alertness and attention span), muscle weakness and increased susceptibility to infections.

As with copper, iron has a dark side. Biologically, it exists in two states: ferrous and ferric. Free iron (not bound to protein structure) in the ferrous state is a powerful generator of destructive oxygen radicals. Free iron is terribly toxic to living cells. There are rare pathological conditions characterized by an excessive amount of free iron in the body. Hemochromatosis is a genetic disorder wherein there are excess deposits of iron in the liver, heart, pancreas, skin and other organs, all of which are subject to serious damage from the toxic oxygen radicals generated by free iron. Fortunately, iron is usually bound very tightly to biological structures; thus most of us are exposed to very little free iron.

Iron is enormously important in human health.

II. Claims

POSITIVE:
1) Prevents and cures iron-deficiency and pernicious anemia; 2) antioxidant; 3) anticarcinogenic; 4) stimulates immunity; 5) boosts physical performance; 6) prevents learning disorders in children.

NEGATIVE:
1) Promotes oxidation; 2) depresses immunity; 3) toxic after prolonged use; 4) destroys vitamin E.

III. Evidence

RELATED TO POSITIVE CLAIMS:

1) Prevents and cures iron-deficiency and pernicious anemia—
Clearly, iron is necessary to prevent iron-deficiency anemia; it is *the* treatment for that disorder. Some, however, claim that supplemental iron is also effective in the treatment of *pernicious* anemia. This is not so. These are two different conditions.

It should be understood that anemia is not a disease. It is a sign of the presence of disease process. Anemia (literally, without blood) refers to a significant decrease in the number of red blood cells. The body normally has about 25 trillion red blood cells (more in men than in women). Hemoglobin, the protein pigment that gives blood its color (red if oxygenated, blue if not), comprises about 30 percent of the red blood cell. This protein is responsible for the carriage of oxygen in the blood to the tissue. When the red-blood-cell count falls, so does the hemoglobin content and the oxygen-carrying capacity of the blood. Decreased oxygenation of tissues leads to decreased energy production with all its attendant symptoms of fatigue, muscle weakness and the like. Significant anemia occurs when the red-blood-cell count falls below about 15 trillion (in adults).

Anemia occurs in three situations: decreased production of red blood cells, abnormal red-blood-cell destruction, or bleeding. Abnormalities in the production of red blood cells occur either because of a defect in the synthesis of the major protein of the cell, hemoglobin, or because of a defect in the synthesis of DNA. A defect in the synthesis of hemoglobin produces a small, pale-appearing cell. This is the case with iron deficiency. When DNA synthesis is interfered with, the cell is usually very large and not pale-appearing. This is what occurs with pernicious anemia, which is thought to be an autoimmune disorder affecting the stomach and producing a vitamin B_{12} deficiency. The treatment of *pernicious* anemia is not with iron but with B_{12}.

2) Antioxidant—Iron is involved in the structure of certain enzymes that protect against oxidant damage: catalase, peroxidase and iron superoxide dismutase. Catalase is found in humans, especially in red blood cells. Iron-containing peroxidases are not very abundant in humans, though hemoglobin itself has a small amount of peroxidase activity. Iron-containing superoxide dismutase is found in bacteria but not in humans. Iron defiency does produce a decrease in catalase activity (*Federation Proceedings, Federation of the American Society for Experimental Biology*, Abstract No. 5215, Apr. 1983, p. 1182), and the red blood cells of patients with the rare disorder acatalasemia (lack of catalase activity) do suffer greater oxidant damage than do normal red cells. Iron appears to play an antioxidant role, but much more research is needed to determine its nature and importance.

3) Anticarcinogenic—Iron deficiency has been associated with the Plummer-Vinson syndrome. In this condition, there is dif-

ficulty swallowing solid food because of a thin, weblike membrane that grows across the upper passageway of the esophagus (gullet). People with this problem are at increased risk of cancer of the esophagus and stomach. This syndrome has been fairly common in Sweden, but iron supplementation has now practically eliminated it (*Cancer Research*, 35:3308, 1975).

In experimental research, iron deficiency has been found to accelerate chemical tumor induction in rats (*Advances in Experimental Medicine and Biology*, 91:229, 1978), though the significance, if any, of this for humans remains to be demonstrated.

Evidence of an anticancer role for iron remains meager. Long-term iron deficiency appears to increase the risk of cancer of the esophagus and stomach in patients with Plummer-Vinson syndrome. On the flip side of the coin, there is no evidence that long-term oral use of iron is associated with an increased incidence of cancer.

4) Stimulates immunity—Resistance to infection depends mainly on the function of the white blood cells, particularly the lymphocytes and the neutrophils. Candida, a pathogenic yeast infection of the skin and mucous membranes, and herpes-simplex infections are more common in patients who are iron deficient (*Journal of Infectious Diseases*, 131:44, 1975; *Iron Metabolism*, Ciba Foundation Symposium No. 51:249, Elsevier, Amsterdam, 1977). Immune responses to skin tests, total lymphocyte numbers and some other indicators of healthy immunity have been shown to decrease in patients with iron deficiency (*Nutrition Research*, 2:721, 1982; *Journal of Clinical Nutrition*, 35:442, 1982).

There is little, if any, effect of iron deficiency on the production of immunoglobulins (B-lymphocyte function). That iron deficiency affects the T-lymphocyte arm of the immune system may have something to do with an enzyme called ribonucleotide reductase. This iron-requiring enzyme is essential for the synthesis of DNA. Decreased activity of this enzyme, due to iron deficiency, could lead to diminished T-cell production and thus impair cell-mediated immune response.

Iron deficiency is also known to impair intracellular killing of bacteria. Certain white blood cells (neutrophils) have iron-requiring proteins that, by generating toxic oxygen radicals, kill bacteria. This is one of the beneficial roles of oxygen radicals.

These proteins are lactoferrin and cytochrome b. Another enzyme that requires iron is myeloperoxidase; it kills bacteria by generating iodine. Lactoferrin is also present in human milk and is thought to confer resistance to infection in nursing infants. Iron deficiencies can interfere with all of these important enzymes.

In summary, it appears that iron plays an important role in cellular immunity and in bacterial killing.

5) Boosts physical performance—Muscle weakness and decreased exercise tolerance, two rather nonspecific symptoms, are frequently associated with iron-deficiency anemia. Remarkably, the degree of disability to perform muscular work is often much greater than would be expected from the degree of anemia present. In fact, these symptoms can occur when there is iron deficiency but no anemia and can be resolved when the iron deficiency is corrected (*British Journal of Haematology*, 41:365, 1979).

From my own clinical experience, I have observed that not only does skeletal-muscle weakness appear out of proportion to the degree of anemia, but cardiac-muscle performance does as well, suggesting that iron deficiency impacts in ways that are in addition to and perhaps independent of the anemia. Frequently, patients with preexisting coronary heart disease develop symptoms of heart failure (shortness of breath, edema) when they develop an iron deficiency (usually from internal bleeding or frequent blood drawing) that is similarly out of proportion with the degree of their anemia.

Iron plays several roles in biological energy production: the transfer of oxygen to tissues by hemoglobin and myoglobin; the transfer of electrons, by means of the cytochromes and cytochrome oxidase in the metabolic furnaces of the cells, to oxygen; the activation of enzymes that oxidize foodstuffs to produce energy; the transport of fatty acids into the metabolic furnaces via involvement with carnitine (fatty acids are the major source of energy in muscle, and carnitine, discussed later in this book, requires iron for its synthesis).

The decrease in oxygen transport to muscle seen in iron-deficiency anemia results in decreased muscular activity since oxygen is necessary for energy production. But it has been demonstrated that iron-deficient animals still often exhibit muscle weakness even when there is no apparent anemia (*Journal of Clinical Investigation*, 58:447, 1976).

It can be concluded that muscular performance (skeletal and cardiac) depends upon adequate availability of iron. Even iron deficiencies that do not produce anemia can affect this performance. More research is needed and justified to help fully clarify the role of iron—and perhaps carnitine—in muscular performance.

6) Prevents learning disorders in children—Iron-deficiency anemia has been implicated in emotional, social and learning difficulties in infants, adolescents and adults. Iron-deficient infants are often irritable and lack interest in their surroundings. Oski and Honig (*Journal of Pediatrics*, 92:21, 1978) reported abnormal reactivity in infants with iron-deficiency anemia and demonstrated improvement after treatment with iron supplements. Lozoff and co-workers (*Iron Deficiency: Brain Biochemistry and Behavior*, Raven Press, New York, 1982, p. 183) clearly showed differences in behavior between iron-deficient and iron-sufficient infants. The anemic infants were less responsive, more tense, less active and more fearful than the nonanemic infants. However, the one week of oral-iron treatment used in this trial proved insufficient to change this behavior. Walter et al. (*Journal of Pediatrics*, 102:519, 1983) also report behavioral differences between iron-sufficient and iron-deficient infants. In this study, two weeks of oral-iron therapy succeeded in removing these differences. This study is particularly interesting because the same behavioral abnormalities were found in infants with iron-deficiency anemia and in infants with iron deficiency but no anemia, indicating that the abnormalities are not simply a matter of decreased oxygen to the brain.

There is mounting evidence that iron deficiency affects infant behavior. And since iron deficiency is a significant problem in infants, particularly disadvantaged infants, it is imperative that the nature of the relation between iron deficiency and behavioral problems of infants be studied and corrected. Some of the behavioral alterations observed in iron deficiency may be related to the synthesis or action of such brain molecules as serotonin, dopamine and noradrenalin, all of which are thought to play crucial roles in behavior.

RELATED TO NEGATIVE CLAIMS:

1) Promotes oxidation—It has been argued that iron can generate free radicals that can cause genetic mutations, atherosclerotic plaques and cancer. Blake and co-workers (*Lancet*, 2:1142, 1981) hypothesize that iron in the membranes of the joints of patients with rheumatoid arthritis contributes to this disease by its generation of free radicals and subsequent lipid peroxidation. Sullivan (*Lancet*, 1:1293, 1981) postulates that the greater incidence of coronary heart disease in men, compared to women, in affluent societies is due to higher levels of stored iron in men.

That iron can generate free radicals is well known. *Unbound* iron in the ferrous (or "plus two") state is a potent generator of hydroxyl radicals, which can be very destructive to cells. However, unbound iron occurs only under certain conditions. Patients with hemochromatosis, a genetic disorder of excessive iron accumulation, can have a significant quantity of unbound iron in their cells, and this may give rise to extensive damage to liver, heart, pancreas and skin. These genetic disorders, however, are rare. And there is no convincing evidence at present that iron is active in either rheumatoid arthritis or atherosclerotic disease. Most iron we come in contact with is tightly bound to protein and does not generate dangerous free radicals.

2) Depresses immunity—Though iron deficiency is usually associated with decreased resistance to infection, there are a few reports (see, for example, *American Journal of Clinical Nutrition*, 31:660, 1978) contending just the opposite, that iron deficiency decreases *susceptibility* to infection. However, except under rare circumstances (such as described in *Lancet*, 2:325, 1974) there is little reason to expect iron to depress immunity. People on long-term iron supplementation are *not* noted for problems with infection.

3) Toxic after prolonged use—Prolonged administration of iron supplements very rarely causes iron overload (Beutler, *Modern Nutrition in Health and Disease*, Lea and Febiger, Philadelphia, 1980, p. 324). It is possible that in those situations where iron overload does occur, the individual has the predisposition for excessive iron absorption called hemochromatosis. Iron sup-

plements are widely used in the United States, and reports of toxicity from iron overload are very rare.

4) Destroys vitamin E—We've known about an iron/vitamin E connection for some time. Ferric chloride, a form of iron, converts vitamin E to an inactive substance. Ferric chloride has also been shown to make rats infertile, apparently by inactivating vitamin E; fertility was restored by the addition of more vitamin E to the diet. A number of additional reports also document an antagonism between *inorganic* iron and vitamin E (see, for example, *British Journal of Experimental Pathology*, 39:59, 1958).

IV. Recommendations

A) SUGGESTED INTAKE: Iron requirements and Recommended Dietary Allowances are shown in Table 1 (see page 158). The average American diet contains 6 milligrams of iron per 1,000 kilocalories. Groups at risk for iron deficiency include infants, adolescents, premenopausal women (especially those on low-calorie diets), pregnant and lactating women, vegetarians and the elderly with poor dietary habits over long periods of time. Iron supplementation is commonly recommended by pediatricians for infants and children at a dose of 10 to 12 milligrams daily (elemental iron). Pregnant and lactating women usually are prescribed 60 milligrams of iron daily. It is wise for adults on low-calorie diets to take 18 milligrams of supplemental iron daily. Adult men who eat well-balanced diets of 2,000 calories or more do not need iron supplements. Elderly persons who feel weak and tired most of the time should see their doctors before starting on iron, since they may be anemic from internal bleeding. Iron itself will do nothing to combat bleeding. In general, I see no reason for adults to consume more than 18 milligrams of iron daily (except during pregnancy or in the event of iron-deficiency anemia, which should be treated by a physician).

B) SOURCE/FORM: The best dietary sources of iron are meat (especially organ meats, such as liver), poultry and fish. Foods with low iron availability include eggs, spinach and many green vegetables. The most bioavailable form of iron, that is, the type

TABLE 1
IRON REQUIREMENTS AND RECOMMENDED
DIETARY ALLOWANCES

AGE (YEARS)	IRON REQUIREMENT[a] (MILLIGRAMS/DAY)	RDA[b] (MILLIGRAMS/DAY)
Infants and children		
0–0.5	0.5–1.5	10
0.5–1	0.5–1.5	15
1–3	0.4–1	15
4–6	0.4–1	10
7–10	0.4–1	10
Males		
11–18	1–2	18
19–50	0.65–1.3	10
51+	0.65–1.3	10
Females		
11–18	1–2.7	18
19–50	0.7–2.3	18
51+	0.6–0.9	10
Pregnant	1.65–3.5	30–60
Lactating		30–60 for 2–3 months after delivery, then 18

a. Iron requirements refer to amount of absorbed iron needed. Estimates taken from Beutler, *Modern Nutrition in Health and Disease*, eds. Goodhart and Shils, Lea and Febiger, Philadelphia, 1980.

b. Recommended Dietary Allowance (RDA), National Research Council, *Recommended Dietary Allowances*, 1980.
   The values refer to daily food intake. The assumption is made that 10 percent of the iron gets absorbed. Since it is unlikely that a pregnant or lactating woman can get 30 to 60 milligrams of dietary iron daily, supplemental iron is recommended.

that can be most easily absorbed by the body, is heme iron found in meats. Meats, moreover, have a factor that increases the availability of nonheme iron.

There are several iron supplements on the market; these include ferrous sulfate, ferrous fumarate and ferrous gluconate. They all have similar bioavailability. I recommend *ferrous sulfate*, however, because it is the cheapest and is as effective as any of the others. Time-release or enteric-coated products are *not* reliably absorbed; moreover, they usually cost more. Don't waste money on them. Absorption is best if taken between meals. Calcium decreases iron availability, while vitamin C increases it. Some products claim that vitamin B_{12} and folic acid aid in the prevention of iron deficiency. These claims are unfounded.

C) TAKE WITH: (See Part Three for recommendations.)

D) CAUTIONARY NOTE: Iron supplements may cause abdominal pain, diarrhea or constipation and they may color the stool a very dark brown to black. If such symptoms arise and persist, cut back on the amount of supplementation, and in any event, do not exceed the amounts recommended above. Do not take iron supplements at all if you have been diagnosed as having idiopathic hemochromatosis (a tendency toward excessive absorption of iron). Persons with anemia should use supplemental iron according to the prescriptions of their physicians. A complete blood count, including hemoglobin and hematocrit determination, will tell you if you are anemic. To determine if you are iron deficient, the tests used are: serum iron (low in iron deficiency), serum transferrin (normal or elevated in iron deficiency) and serum ferritin (low in iron deficiency).

Magnesium

I. Overview

The primordial oceans on this planet were rich in magnesium and potassium. Sodium rules the seas today, but the waters within our cells remain true to the "primordial soup" from which all life arose, rich in magnesium and potassium. Optimal health depends upon the maintenance of this condition. Magnesium is not a trace mineral but a major entity in our bodies. Most of it is in our bones and in the waters within the cells. Magnesium is absolutely essential for life. It is necessary for every major biological process, including the metabolism of glucose, production of cellular energy, and the synthesis of nucleic acids and protein.

It is also important for the electrical stability of cells, the maintenance of membrane integrity, muscle contraction, nerve conduction and the regulation of vascular tone. It is intimately interlocked, biologically, with calcium. In some reactions, such as the synthesis of nucleic acids and protein, calcium and magnesium are antagonistic. Magnesium is necessary for these processes, while calcium inhibits them. Magnesium and calcium collaborate, however, in the production of the crystal of biological energy, adenosine triphosphate. Magnesium appears to regulate the gate through which calcium enters into cells to switch on such vital functions as the heartbeat.

Magnesium deficiency is characterized by loss of appetite, nausea, vomiting, diarrhea, confusion, tremors, loss of coordination and, occasionally, fatal convulsions. Magnesium deficiency is sometimes associated with concurrent deficiencies of calcium and potassium.

It is becoming increasingly evident that marginal magnesium deficiency is very common. Particularly vulnerable groups include the elderly, those on low-calorie diets, diabetics, those taking diuretics and digitalis preparations, consumers of alcohol, pregnant women, and people who exercise regularly and strenuously (*Journal of Applied Physiology*, 29:449, 1970; *Aviation, Space and Environmental Medicine*, 46:709, 1975). The adequacy of our dietary magnesium has been questioned (*American Journal of Clinical Nutrition*, 14:342, 1964). It is now recognized that even marginal magnesium deficiency can predispose one to life-threatening cardiac dysrhythmias (disruption of normal heart rhythm). Although it has not been proved, magnesium supplementation may protect against the plague of Western civilization—ischemic heart disease (oxygen starvation of heart muscle caused by spasms or narrowing and clogging of the arteries leading to the heart).

Magnesium supplementation appears poised to play a key role in preventive medicine.

II. Claims

POSITIVE:
1) Protective against cardiovascular disease and helpful in the treatment of high blood pressure; 2) beneficial in the treatment of the premenstrual syndrome; 3) helps prevent kidney stones and gallstones; 4) useful in the treatment of prostate problems; 5) useful in the treatment of polio; 6) aids in fighting depression;

7) effective in the treatment of convulsions in pregnant women and prevents premature labor; 8) beneficial in the treatment of neuromuscular and nervous disorders; 9) effective in the treatment of diarrhea, vomiting and indigestion.

NEGATIVE:
1) Toxic.

III. Evidence

RELATED TO POSITIVE CLAIMS:

1) Protective against cardiovascular disease and helpful in the treatment of high blood pressure—Epidemiological studies suggest that the death rate from ischemic heart disease is increased in areas with soft, as opposed to hard, water (*British Medical Bulletin*, 27:21, 1971). Hard water contains both magnesium and calcium. However, it is the view of Seelig (*American Journal of Clinical Nutrition*, 27:59, 1974) that magnesium is the more important factor in the protection against ischemic heart disease. Seelig has presented evidence that Western diet is deficient in magnesium and proposes that this may underlie the very high incidence of cardiovascular disease in Western nations, especially among men. Findings have conflicted to some extent (*Circulation*, 63:247A, 1981), but Seelig's hypothesis certainly warrants further investigation, particularly in view of recent findings that magnesium does indeed play an extremely important role in the maintenance of the electrical and physical integrity of heart muscle.

One of the causes of ischemic heart disease, wherein the coronary arteries fail to provide all of the oxygen that the heart demands, is spasm in the smooth muscles of the artery walls. It seems reasonable to postulate that inadequate magnesium may make the coronary arteries more susceptible to muscle spasm. Too little magnesium may mean too much calcium, and the toxic effects of calcium ions could potentiate spasm. The same applies to the muscular activity of the heart itself. Calcium is crucial for this activity, but if too much ionic calcium enters the heart cells (because the "gatekeeper," magnesium, is in short supply) then the effect can be disruptive, introducing toxic, killing forms of oxygen. This may be at the very root of heart-tissue death and thus of myocardial infarction (heart attack). A magnesium-calcium imbalance may not only predispose to cardiovascular disease but may also make repair very difficult. Once calcium has the upper hand its natural antagonism to magnesium makes it all the more difficult for the latter to promote the nucleic acid and protein syntheses that are at the literal heart, in this case, of the mending process.

More research will have to be done before it can legitimately be claimed that magnesium supplementation is of benefit in ischemic heart disease. But we do know that magnesium deficiency predisposes humans to potentially fatal disruptions of normal cardiac rhythm (cardiac dysrhythmia). Iseri and co-workers (*Western Journal of Medicine*, 138:823, 1983) have successfully treated ventricular dysrhythmias with magnesium. These disorders had not been improved by conventional drug therapy. Remarkably, the levels of magnesium in the blood of these patients were normal. That *cellular* magnesium deficiency can exist in the context of normal blood magnesium levels, however, has been demonstrated by Cohen and Kitzes (*Journal of American Medical Association*, 249:2808, 1983). They report successful treatment (with magnesium) of cardiac-dysrhythmia patients taking diuretics and digitalis. Cellular (lymphocyte) levels of magnesium were depleted in these patients even though their blood levels were normal. The cellular measure is a far more accurate gauge and should be employed more often, especially when dealing with patients on diuretics and digitalis, both of which are known to diminish magnesium levels (*British Medical Journal*, 285:1377, 1982).

Dyckner and Wester (*British Medical Journal*, 286:1847, 1983), meanwhile, report that patients with essential hypertension have better control of their blood pressure when given magnesium supplementation. These patients are also taking diuretics.

More research is definitely warranted.

2) Beneficial in the treatment of the premenstrual syndrome—This syndrome refers to cyclic symptoms experienced by women during their reproductive years; these symptoms may include anxiety, irritability, mood swings, breast tenderness, fatigue, dizziness, headache, etc. Abraham (*Journal of Reproductive Medicine*, 28:446, 1983) believes that magnesium, zinc and some vitamin deficiencies play a central role in this syndrome. He

reasons that refined sugars and high dairy-product intake decrease magnesium absorption and that the resulting deficiency leads to a decreased synthesis of the brain neurotransmitter dopamine, which, in turn, causes an imbalance in other brain chemicals. This and other disruptions, he believes, cause the symptoms of premenstrual syndrome. Goei and Abraham (*Journal of Reproductive Medicine*, 28:527, 1983) report that vitamin and mineral supplementation, including magnesium, provided some measurable relief for some women with this syndrome. The trial was not placebo-controlled.

There are insufficient data at present to substantiate or refute this claim. More research will have to be done.

3) Helps prevent kidney stones and gallstones—Two studies report the beneficial effect of magnesium supplementation in the prevention of recurrent calcium-oxalate stones. One study (*American Journal of Clinical Nutrition*, 20:399, 1967) used 200 milligrams daily of magnesium oxide plus 10 milligrams daily of vitamin B_6. In the second study (*Journal of Urology*, 112:509, 1974) magnesium was used alone—in the amount of 300 milligrams of magnesium oxide daily. The current evidence suggests that magnesium supplementation is effective in preventing calcium-oxalate stones in people who have this recurrent problem. (It is presently estimated that about one million Americans now living will die from causes related to kidney stones, the causes of which remain obscure.) Gallstones, in contrast to kidney stones, only rarely contain calcium; there is no evidence that magnesium either prevents or is useful in the treatment of gallstones.

4) Useful in the treatment of prostate problems—There is no evidence to support this claim.

5) Useful in the treatment of polio—There is no evidence to support this claim.

6) Aids in fighting depression—Depression is one of the most complex human phenomena. It is characterized by sleep disturbances, loss of interest in the world, guilty feelings, loss of energy, inability to concentrate, decreased appetite for food (and often for all of life), diminished psychomotor activity and occasionally by suicidal thoughts. Depression is not uncommon,

especially in the elderly, and is one of the most difficult challenges faced by the physician. We still know very little about the bases of depression. There is no evidence as yet that magnesium can play any useful role in the treatment of depression. Almost no research has been done in this context, but we do know that magnesium is involved in the synthesis of some of the brain neurotransmitters. We also know that marginal magnesium deficiency increases with age. The preliminary data on magnesium in the treatment of premenstrual syndrome (see discussion above) at least suggest that supplementary magnesium might have some favorable effect on some of the neurotransmitters. Here is an area that needs more research.

7) Effective in the treatment of convulsions in pregnant women and prevents premature labor—There is a very threatening syndrome that occasionally occurs during pregnancy called pre-eclampsia/eclampsia. Preeclampsia is characterized by high blood pressure, swelling of the body (sometimes the entire body) and the finding of protein in the urine. Preeclampsia can develop into the far more serious eclampsia, in which convulsions, coma and even death can occur. Intravenous magnesium (magnesium sulfate) has been used successfully for many years in the treatment of this syndrome. The mechanism by which magnesium works in this case is unknown. It is possible, however, that women who develop this disorder have a marginal magnesium deficiency. If there is not enough magnesium in the body to regulate the flow of calcium into the cells, an excess of calcium may cause constriction of the smooth muscles in blood vessels and in the uterus, accounting for at least part of the syndrome. A recent report (*American Journal of Obstetrics and Gynecology*, 147:277, 1983) showed intravenous magnesium sulfate to be beneficial in the inhibition of premature labor. Prematurity is the single greatest cause of disease and death in the newborn. Magnesium may, in this instance, be helping to maintain the muscle of the uterus in a relaxed condition until the fetus is fully ready to enter the outside world. More research is clearly called for.

8) Beneficial in the treatment of neuromuscular and nervous disorders—It is true that in clear-cut cases of magnesium deficiency, muscle weakness, tremors and various movement disorders may arise that can be resolved with supplemental

magnesium. There is no evidence, however, that magnesium supplements can be of benefit in these disorders in individuals not suffering from severe magnesium deficiency.

9) Effective in the treatment of diarrhea, vomiting and indigestion—Loss of appetite, nausea, vomiting and diarrhea are, in fact, among the early symptoms of magnesium deficiency. However, these symptoms are so general that they could be—and usually are—related to a multitude of other factors. Most of the magnesium products on the market do not have an antidiarrhea effect but actually *cause* diarrhea. Such products as Phillips' Milk of Magnesia and Haley's M-O, both of which contain magnesium hydroxide, are sold as laxatives in the treatment of constipation. Some of the magnesium-containing antacids on the market, though they help with indigestion, also can cause diarrhea.

RELATED TO NEGATIVE CLAIMS:

1) Toxic—There are two situations in which increasing magnesium intake is not desirable. Magnesium should not be administered to patients with severely decreased renal (kidney) function and in those with high-grade atrioventricular blocks or bifascicular blocks. Magnesium, in these instances, could slow down the heart rate and lead to depression of neuromuscular function and even to respiratory depression. Paradoxically, many of the cardiac patients with these blocks may be suffering from marginal magnesium deficiency, in part because they often use diuretics and the heart drug digitalis. If such patients are fitted with artificial pacemakers, magnesium supplementation will not present the same risks—but all such patients should consult with their physicians before taking any magnesium supplements. They should also be careful about using over-the-counter magnesium-containing antacids and laxatives.

Except in the conditions described above, there is no evidence that magnesium supplements are harmful to people. Diarrhea may be avoided by taking magnesium in the form of magnesium gluconate.

IV. Recommendations

A) SUGGESTED INTAKE: The National Research Council recommends a daily allowance of 350 milligrams of magnesium for men and 300 milligrams for women. An additional allowance of 150 milligrams daily is recommended for pregnant and lactating (nursing) women. The magnesium content of the average American diet is estimated at 120 milligrams per 1,000 kilocalories. Dietary intake of magnesium may be inadequate in large segments of the population. It is prudent to take supplementary magnesium. I recommend a supplementary intake of 200 to 400 milligrams daily. Those who may, in particular, benefit from such supplementation include the elderly, those on low-calorie diets, diabetics, people taking diuretics and digitalis preparations (though the latter should consult their doctors before taking any supplements), consumers of alcohol, pregnant women, and those who indulge in regular and strenuous exercise.

B) SOURCE/FORM: Foods rich in magnesium include meats, seafoods, green vegetables and dairy products. Supplementary forms include magnesium oxide, magnesium carbonate, magnesium hydroxide and magnesium gluconate. I recommend magnesium gluconate because it seldom produces diarrhea. Magnesium oxide and magnesium hydroxide, on the other hand, often do cause diarrhea. Magnesium carbonate is not recommended because it is not easily absorbed.

C) TAKE WITH: Best if incorporated into a well-balanced vitamin/mineral preparation (See Part Three for more specific recommendations.)

D) CAUTIONARY NOTE: People with renal failure and high-grade atrioventricular blocks should not take supplementary magnesium. (See Evidence section, Related to Negative Claims, for details.) Patients with high-grade heart blocks may take supplementary magnesium if they have artificial pacemakers, though they should first consult with their physicians and follow their instructions. Note that the conventional test for magnesium deficiency—a measure of blood levels of this mineral—*does not* necessarily reflect actual body stores of magnesium. The best test—not widely available—analyzes magnesium levels in *lymphocytes* (white blood cells).

Manganese

I. Overview

Oxygen was absent from the atmosphere when the earth was newly born about four and a half billion years ago and did not appear until about two and a half billion years later. At that time the blue-green algae (a type of bacteria) came into being and were able to split water into oxygen by using the energy of the sun. It was manganese that made this possible. Today, one of manganese's principal roles is that of *anti*oxidant and, as such, may help protect humans from toxic oxygen forms.

Manganese, for the most part, however, remains an enigma with respect to its possible roles in human biology. Manganese-deficiency states are known in animals (these include defective growth and neurological disorders) but have not been documented in man. There is one report of what may be such a deficiency in man. Doisy (*Trace Element Metabolism in Animals*, University Park Press, Baltimore, 1974) apparently produced manganese deficiency in a patient who was maintained for four months on a manganese-deficient diet and who simultaneously was given magnesium-containing antacids. The symptoms included: decrease in serum cholesterol, impaired blood clotting, reddening of his black hair and beard, slowed growth of hair and nails, and scaly dermatitis. Doisy suggests that in man this element functions in both glycoprotein synthesis (some of the clotting factors are protein with carbohydrates attached to them) and cholesterol synthesis.

A fascinating pathological state in man is manganese intoxication, an understanding of which may eventually yield important clues regarding the role of manganese in the human body. Dietary manganese has low toxicity, but mine workers exposed to high concentrations of manganese dust develop what is known in the mining villages of northern Chile, where this disorder is most common, as "*locura manganica*," or manganese madness. The early stage of this disorder is marked by unaccountable laughter, heightened sexuality, impulsiveness, inability to fall asleep, delusions and hallucinations. This manic state is followed by a state of deep depression, which is distinguished by slow speech, impotence and inability to stay awake. In the final stage of the disease process, symptoms similar to those of

Parkinson's disease are observed. Parkinson's is a degenerative disease of the brain resulting from the loss of dopamine-containing cells. The treatment is a drug called L-dopa, which the brain can convert to dopamine. L-dopa is also the treatment of the chronic stage of manganese poisoning.

Although to this date we do not know the unique functions of manganese in human biology, what we do know suggests that it is essential. It is conceivable that this element is *so* important that nature has invented ways to ensure that manganese-deficiency states do not occur or almost never occur. Such mechanisms *may* include the ability of magnesium to substitute for manganese in many biochemical reactions, thus sparing manganese when its stores are low. With regard to the aging process, manganese's probable role as an antioxidant is interesting. In this regard, it is noteworthy that *all* tumors examined to date have diminished amounts of the manganese-containing superoxide-dismutase enzyme (*Cancer Research*, 39:1141, 1979). This provides a hint, but certainly not proof, that manganese deficiency may play a role in degenerative processes in humans. Manganese has a fascinating past; I suspect it has a promising future.

II. Claims

POSITIVE:
1) Antioxidant; 2) important for the normal functioning of the brain and effective in the treatment of schizophrenia and some nervous disorders; 3) necessary for reproduction; 4) needed for normal bone structure and helpful in the treatment of osteoarthritis; 5) necessary for normal glucose metabolism and beneficial in the treatment of diabetes mellitus; 6) miscellaneous.

NEGATIVE:
1) Toxic.

III. Evidence

RELATED TO POSITIVE CLAIMS:

1) Antioxidant—Donaldson and co-workers (*Canadian Journal of Physiology and Pharmacology*, 60:1398, 1982) propose that all

of the symptoms of manganese neurotoxicity can be explained by the antioxidant and prooxidant (oxidant-promoting) properties of the element. Manganese can exist in different forms (different valence states or combining states); divalent manganese is a scavenger of oxygen free radicals, in short, an antioxidant. Some higher valence states, however, such as trivalent manganese, are prooxidants and as such can lead to the generation of free radicals and resulting damage. The authors postulate that the manganese that is normally present in the brain is of the favorable variety and that it uniquely counteracts oxidant damage when everything is operating as it should, and thus protects against degenerative neurological diseases. An additional antioxidant role may be played by the enzyme manganese superoxide dismutase; the protection here would be at the cellular level thoughout the body. More research will have to be done before any authoritative conclusions can be reached with respect to manganese's antioxidant properties in humans.

2) Important for the normal functioning of the brain and effective in the treatment of schizophrenia and some nervous disorders—See also discussion above. Manganese appears to be involved in the synthesis of the neurotransmitter dopamine in the brain (*Advances in Neurology*, 5:235, 1974), although more research will have to be done before this role is convincingly established. There are anecdotal reports of the effectiveness of manganese in the treatment of schizophrenia. Pfeiffer (*Zinc and Other Micro-Nutrients*, Keats, New Canaan, Conn., 1978) has been arguing for years that copper contributes to certain types of schizophrenia. He believes that manganese, as well as zinc, decreases dietary copper absorption (see analysis of copper elsewhere in this book) and in so doing aids in the treatment of schizophrenia. There are no controlled studies to substantiate any of this. There is no proof that copper plays a role in any form of schizophrenia and no evidence that manganese lowers copper levels in humans, although zinc certainly can do this. (See discussion of zinc elsewhere in this book.) There are also reports (R. A. Kunin, *Mega-Nutrition*, New American Library, New York, 1981) that manganese can be useful in the treatment of tardive dyskinesia, a neurological disorder caused by neuroleptic drugs (major tranquilizers). These reports are anecdotal.

3) Necessary for reproduction—Manganese-deficient animals sometimes exhibit reproductive difficulties; this may be due to the requirement for manganese in the synthesis of cholesterol, which is itself the precursor of the sex steroids. Manganese may have this function in humans, but this has not been demonstrated to date.

4) Needed for normal bone structure and helpful in the treatment of osteoarthritis—Skeletal abnormalities have been observed in manganese-deficient animals and have been linked to a reduction in the synthesis of mucopolysaccharides, which make up the matrix of the cartilage at the ends of bones (within which bone formation takes place). Manganese is involved in this synthesis in animals and may play a similar, though yet unestablished, role in humans.

Frank (*Nucleic Acid and Antioxidant Therapy of Aging and Degeneration*, Rainstone Publishing, New York, 1977) proposed that manganese should be useful in the treatment of osteoarthritis, a degenerative joint disease characterized by a loss of joint cartilage and hypertrophy (overgrowth) of bone. Frank reasoned that if manganese were involved in mucopolysaccharide formation, then manganese may function to repair worn-out cartilage. This is an untested hypothesis, though there are a few anecdotal reports claiming that manganese is effective in the treatment of osteoarthritis. The claims here are not unreasonable and deserve some investigation.

5) Necessary for normal glucose metabolism and beneficial in the treatment of diabetes mellitus—Manganese deficiency in animals does lead to decreased glucose tolerance (the ability to metabolize this sugar); however, there is *no* evidence that this is true in humans, and there are no studies showing manganese to be useful in the treatment of any form of human diabetes.

6) Miscellaneous—There is no evidence whatever for claims that manganese is important for the formation of thyroid hormone, that it promotes maternal instincts, that it is useful in the treatment of multiple sclerosis and myasthenia gravis, that it helps overcome dizziness and eliminate stress, fatigue, absent-mindedness and irritability.

RELATED TO NEGATIVE CLAIMS:

1) Toxic—The toxicity of dietary manganese is low. Inhaled manganese dust can, as explained in the Overview, cause serious neurological disease. A matter of concern is the recent practice of adding manganese as an antiknock agent in automobile fuel (to replace lead). The use of these manganese compounds has not yet caused dangerous levels of manganese air pollution, but this could change. The situation should be carefully monitored and studied. "Manganese madness" is a very serious matter.

IV. Recommendations

A) SUGGESTED INTAKE: Optimal manganese intake is unknown. The National Research Council lists the estimated safe and adequate daily dietary intake of manganese for adults at 2.5 to 5 milligrams. Up to 10 milligrams daily are considered safe. High dietary magnesium, calcium and phosphate may decrease the absorption of manganese. So may antacids and laxatives that contain magnesium. Given the low toxicity of manganese and the potentially important role that it plays in human health, I believe it is prudent to incorporate 5 milligrams daily (adults) in one's supplement program. Doses higher than 10 milligrams daily are not recommended.

B) SOURCE/FORM: The best dietary sources of manganese include whole grains and nuts. Fruits and green vegetables contain moderate amounts, content depending upon the soil in which the crops were grown. The more alkaline the soil the less manganese there will be in the food. Manganese is concentrated in the bran of grains, which is removed during processing. Organ meats and shellfish are additional good sources of this element. The most common supplementary forms of manganese are manganese sulfate and manganese gluconate. They both deliver about the same amount of manganese to the body; the sulfate is usually less expensive.

C) TAKE WITH: Best incorporated into a well-balanced vitamin/mineral "insurance" formula; see Part Three.

D) NOTE: There is no routine test presently available to assess individual manganese status. Promising tests, which may become available in the future, include whole-blood analysis and mitochondrial manganese superoxide-dismutase levels.

Molybdenum

I. Overview

Although molybdenum is a relative newcomer on the supplement scene, it is already gathering quite a colorful history. Compounds of molybdenum are among the scarcer constituents of the earth's crust. This scarcity has been associated with one of the world's highest incidences of esophageal cancer—in an area of China. The discrepancy between its rarity in the earth and its abundance in living things has been used in support of a postulate that life on this planet was seeded by microorganisms sent by some form of intelligent life on another planet rich in this element (Crick and Orgel, *Icarus*, 19:341, 1973).

Molybdenum is a trace mineral that is found in all tissues of the human body and is required for the activity of several enzymes. Only recently has a human deficiency state for molybdenum been described. Abumrad and co-workers (*American Journal of Clinical Nutrition*, 34:2551, 1981) described a patient fed intravenously who became intolerant of the sulfur-containing amino acids and developed a fast heartbeat, increased rate of breathing, visual problems and finally became comatose. This patient was found to have high blood sulfite levels. After molybdenum (as ammonium molybdate) was added to the intravenous feeding solution, the patient improved and the sulfite level returned to normal. At least from this isolated case it appears that the deleterious effects of molybdenum deficiency are due to the accumulation of sulfite, which is toxic to the nervous system. There have been no other reports of molybdenum deficiency.

Sulfiting agents are extensively used for the preservation of foods and drugs. These are not harmless substances and can cause nausea, diarrhea, acute asthma attacks, loss of consciousness and even death in certain individuals (FDA *Drug Bulletin*, 13, 1983). Bisulfite, itself, can destroy vitamin B_1. Ideally, less toxic substances should be substituted. These substances are probably detoxified in the body by means of the molybdenum-activated enzyme sulfite oxidase. Thus, in this capacity, molybdenum is a detoxifier of potentially hazardous substances we all come in contact with almost daily.

Molybdenum may also play a useful antioxidant role. Uric acid has been shown to be a powerful antioxidant and a scavenger of singlet oxygen and hydroxyl radicals (*Proceedings of the National Academy of Sciences*, 78:6858, 1981). Toxicity of oxygen radicals is thought to be a major factor in degenerative diseases and aging. Uric acid is produced by the molybdenum-activated enzyme xanthine oxidase. Most clinicians see uric acid as, at best, a useless and, at worst, a very destructive molecule in that it can cause gouty arthritis. Biological phenomena, however, often have two sides, as is the case here. Conceivably, an optimal uric-acid level (maybe just short of the point where it begins to cause problems) is essential for optimal health and to slow down the wear and tear of aging. If this is true, then molybdenum does indeed enter the realm of useful antioxidants.

All signs point toward the essentiality of molybdenum for optimal health and life-span.

II. Claims

POSITIVE:
1) Protective against cancer; 2) protects teeth; 3) prevents sexual impotence; 4) prevents anemia and mobilizes iron.

NEGATIVE:
1) Toxic.

III. Evidence

RELATED TO POSITIVE CLAIMS:

1) Protective against cancer—To me, one of the most fascinating programs in the *Nova* television series was "The Cancer Detectives of Lin Xian." Lin Xian is a small region (twenty miles square) in Honan Province in north China (see *Chinese Medical Journal* 1:167–183, 1975), which was documented to have the highest incidence of esophageal cancer in the world. As a result

of outstanding scientific investigation, it was determined that the soil in this area was markedly deficient in molybdenum. In order for nitrates in the soil to be reduced to nitrogenous substances (amines) necessary for plant nutrition, a molybdenum-activated enzyme called nitrate reductase (found in nitrogen-fixing bacteria) is required. Molybdenum deficiency decreases the activity of this enzyme, and, instead of being converted to amines, the nitrates get transformed to nitrosamines, known cancer-causing substances. The people of Lin Xian were also deficient in vitamin C, which has been shown to convert nitrosamines to less toxic forms and thus protect us, to some extent, against them. Armed with this knowledge, the Chinese have now enriched the soil with molybdenum, and the inhabitants of Lin Xian are now taking supplemental vitamin C. As a result, the incidence of esophageal cancer may be declining for the first time in more than two thousand years (*Chinese Medical Journal*, 1:167, 1975, and *Cancer Research*, 40:2633, 1980). Low levels of molybdenum in the soil and a high incidence of esophageal cancer in the Bantu of the Transkei in South Africa have also been reported (*Journal of the National Cancer Institute*, 36:201, 1966).

In experimental work, Luo and colleagues (*Federation Proceedings, Federation of the American Society for Experimental Biology*, 46:928, 1981) report that molybdenum supplementation protected rats from chemical carcinogens.

There is no evidence that supplementary molybdenum intake in humans protects against cancer, but molybdenum enrichment of the soil (especially in areas deficient in molybdenum) may very well do so—by decreasing the amount of nitrosamines and their precursors that we consume.

2) Protects teeth—A California study (*Journal of Dental Research*, 50:74, 1971) found no difference in the prevalence of cavities among children with high and low intakes of molybdenum. A British study did find a difference—a 20 percent lower incidence of cavities among children with high molybdenum intake. The study (*Caries Research*, 3:75, 1969) was inconclusive, however, particularly in view of the fact that the children with the higher molybdenum intake were also found to have 34 percent more fluoride in their teeth. These skimpy results do not support a role for molybdenum in the prevention of dental cavities.

3) Prevents sexual impotence—This claim has been made, especially with respect to older males. It is purely anecdotal. No studies exist.

4) Prevents anemia and mobilizes iron—There is no evidence that molybdenum deficiency contributes to anemia in humans. Xanthine oxidase, an enzyme dependent upon molybdenum, may participate in the uptake and release of iron from ferritin (storage form of iron), but its role in this regard is not thought to be significant.

RELATED TO NEGATIVE CLAIMS:

1) Toxic—Molybdenum toxicity has been noted in some animals that consume feed high in this mineral. This is due to the antagonism of molybdenum to copper. Dietary intake of 10 to 15 milligrams of molybdenum daily has been associated with goutlike symptoms; the molybdenum-activated enzyme xanthine oxidase makes uric acid, high levels of which can produce gout. Daily intake of .54 milligrams has been associated with a significant loss of copper (see *Recommended Dietary Allowances*, 9th ed., National Academy of Sciences, Washington, D.C., 1980).

IV. Recommendations

A) SUGGESTED INTAKE: The optimal intake of molybdenum is still uncertain. The National Research Council recommends as safe and adequate 0.15 to 0.5 milligram daily for adults. Dietary intake varies considerably from person to person. This intake, in the American diet, has been estimated at between 0.1 and 0.46 milligram. The daily adult intake should not exceed 0.5 milligram since an intake of 0.54 milligram daily has been associated with a significant urinary loss of copper.

Since I believe molybdenum is essential for optimal health—and since I do recommend copper supplementation (see copper analysis)—I propose that a daily supplement of from 50 to 100 micrograms (not milligrams) of molybdenum may be useful for "insurance" purposes.

B) SOURCE/FORM: Molybdenum is found in meat, grains and legumes. Sodium molybdate is available as a supplement, usually in combination with other vitamins and minerals. Sodium molybdate gives good bioavailability and is the least toxic form of molybdenum. Recently a molybdenum-enriched yeast has come on the market. I see no advantage to taking molybdenum in this form, which is considerably more expensive.

C) TAKE WITH: Best if incorporated into a well-balanced vitamin/mineral formula. (See Part Three for further recommendations.) Specifically, I suggest taking 2 to 3 milligrams of copper daily with molybdenum because of the antagonism of the two.

D) CAUTIONARY NOTE: People with high levels of uric acid and/ or gout should consult their physicians before taking molybdenum supplements.

Selenium

I. Overview

If there are emerging "superstars" among the micronutrients, selenium, despite its once sinister reputation, is undoubtedly one of them. With the possible exceptions of vitamin C and beta-carotene, no other micronutrients have excited as much recent scientific interest. More scientific papers are currently being published on selenium than on any other trace element. This is one of those rare instances in which the often excessive claims of the supplement supermarket may actually not yet have caught up with the findings of science.

Selenium is an essential trace mineral required by the body in *minute* quantities. Recognition of its vital importance in human metabolism was long impeded by its very real toxic potential and by fears of carcinogenicity, fears that have now been largely displaced by evidence suggesting just the opposite—that selenium provides *protection* against a large number of cancers and, indeed, against a broad spectrum of diseases.

Once described as "the most maddening, frustrating, nutritional element," selenium was subject to contradictory findings for decades. One group of investigators, for example, casually noted, in one breath, that selenium could dramatically extend the life-spans of animals (producing the longest-lived laboratory rats in history) but then went on to condemn the element, in the next breath, as the probable carcinogen that ultimately killed the very Methuselahs it had helped create! Eventually, however, it was established that selenium *deficiencies* occur in most warm-blooded animals, giving rise to cataracts, muscular dystrophy, growth depression, liver necrosis, infertility, heart disease, cancer and so on. Veterinarian experience led to officially sanctioned supplementation of animal feeds and helped promote many of the experimental and human epidemiological selenium studies that are yielding the often promising results summarized below.

That selenium is essential for optimal health is now established. Chronic illnesses, such as arteriosclerosis (coronary artery disease, cerebrovascular disease and peripheral vascular disease), cancer, degenerative joint disease (arthritis), cirrhosis and chronic obstructive pulmonary disease (emphysema), comprise the overwhelming majority of our health problems. The evidence is mounting that selenium is protective against certain of these diseases and should assume a pivotal role in preventive medicine.

A common denominator in the etiology of most of the chronic diseases we associate with the aging process is oxidant damage to cellular membranes, nucleic acids and proteins. A crucial enzyme in the defense against oxidant damage is glutathione peroxidase. This enzyme contains selenium (in the form of selenocysteine) at each of its four catalytic sites. Selenium thus plays a crucial role in this important enzyme's antioxidant function. But, in addition, selenium may also decrease platelet aggregation, making it further protective against coronary artery disease, strokes and heart attacks. Its role in the immune system, especially in enhancing cellular immunity, may explain its reported anticarcinogenicity.

What all the major theories of aging (reviewed in Chapter One) have in common is the "wear and tear" of some vital cellular component or function. Accumulation of mutations contributes to the process of aging in the somatic-mutation hypothesis. Orgel's "error-catastrophe" hypothesis states that an accumulation of errors in protein synthesis leads to an ultimately irreversible accumulation of errors and a final, lethal catastrophe—death. Another proposal is that decreased lymphocyte formation accelerates the aging process by predisposing to infection, cancer and degenerative diseases. Lipid peroxidation is thought responsible for some of the changes in hormone production and in the hormone receptors that others believe are central to aging.

Selenium is remarkable in that the best evidence suggests that it can have inhibitory effects on *all* of the major hypothesized aging mechanisms. That it can play a very important role in helping to reduce the incidence of many diseases associated with aging appears certain. Adequate selenium intake is unquestionably necessary if one is to attain optimal health and full life-span potential. Man's ability to extend "maximum life-span" beyond presently defined limits remains unproved; if there *are* micronutrients that can help break the present "life-span barrier," selenium has to be accounted one of the prime contenders.

II. Claims

POSITIVE:
1) Antioxidant; 2) anticarcinogenic; 3) immunostimulant; 4) protective against heart and circulatory diseases; 5) capable of detoxifying heavy metals, various drugs, alcohol, cigarette smoke, peroxidized fats; 6) cosmetically beneficial to the skin; 7) increases male potency and sex drive; 8) anti-inflammatory and thus useful against arthritis and other autoimmune diseases.

NEGATIVE:
1) Highly toxic in even minute doses; 2) mutagenic, i.e., capable of producing potentially harmful mutations in cells; 3) carcinogenic; 4) cannot be effective utilized by the body in supplement form; 5) rendered useless by concurrent intake of vitamin C.

III. Evidence

RELATED TO POSITIVE CLAIMS:

1) Antioxidant—Not in dispute. Refer to Chapter One for discussion of antioxidants and their anti-aging effects.

2) Anticarcinogenic—A large body of epidemiological evidence now exists which suggests that cancer mortality goes up when selenium content of soil and thus of crops goes down. Shamber-

ger and colleagues (*Archives of Environmental Health,* 31:231, 1976) have mapped the selenium content of the various states of the U.S. and have found its distribution highly uneven, with the highest levels in South Dakota and the lowest in Ohio. These researchers have shown that Rapid City, South Dakota, has the lowest overall cancer mortality rate in the nation, while Ohio has a rate nearly double that of South Dakota.

Schrauzer et al. (*Bioinorganic Chemistry,* 7:23, 1977, and 8:303, 1978) have confirmed these studies and extended them to more than twenty other nations: the lower the selenium intake, they found, the higher the incidence of leukemia and cancers of the colon, rectum, pancreas, breast, ovary, prostate, bladder, skin and (in the male) lungs. Venezuela, with its high selenium soil content, has, to cite one example, a mortality rate from cancer of the large intestine less than one-quarter that of the U.S. The low incidence of breast cancer among women in Japan has been attributed to their relatively high selenium intake; Japanese women who emigrate to the U.S., however, have a greatly increased incidence of breast cancer. Both Schrauzer and Shamberger have found consistently higher levels of selenium in the blood of healthy individuals than in the blood of those suffering from many forms of cancer.

Willett and co-workers (*Lancet,* July 16, 1983, p. 130) have perhaps the most recent data on blood levels of selenium and cancer incidence. They too report a higher incidence of cancer —especially gastrointestinal and prostatic—among those with lower levels of selenium.

The National Research Council of the National Academy of Sciences (*Diet, Nutrition and Cancer,* National Academy Press, Washington, D.C., 1982) recently asserted that "a large accumulation of evidence indicates that supplementation of the diet or drinking water with selenium protects against tumors induced by a variety of chemical carcinogens and at least one viral agent." This, of course, was done with laboratory animals.

Experimental evidence has shown that selenium added to food or water in doses of 1 to 4 ppm (parts per million) has significantly reduced the incidence of liver, skin, mammary and colon cancers in various laboratory animals. (See review in *Diet, Nutrition and Cancer* cited above.) In one of these experiments (*Bioinorganic Chemistry,* 8:387, 1978) female mice specially bred to develop spontaneous breast tumors were divided into two groups. The "controls" received normal diet; the "experimentals" were given selenium supplements. Breast cancers occurred, as expected, in 82 percent of the controls but in only 10 percent of the selenium-supplemented experimentals.

Most of these studies have shown cancer-*preventive* effects rather than antitumor effects. Recently, however, Ip (*Cancer Research*, 41:4386, 1981) reported that supplemental selenium can retard the recurrence of rat mammary tumors after they have regressed under the influence of other treatment. Greeder and Milner (*Science*, 209:825, 1980) have reported other selenium-induced antitumor effects.

There is some evidence that selenium deficiency is a significantly growing problem. Various explanatory hypotheses have been put forward. One suggests that because sulfur competes with selenium for uptake in plants, increased sulfur-dioxide fall-out and "acid rain" may be contributing to selenium loss.

Selenium's anticancer mechanisms are not yet well understood. Some research suggests that selenium affects enzymatic processes that may inhibit the activation of some carcinogens. Other research indicates that selenium may increase the efficiency of DNA repair mechanisms in the wake of carcinogenic damage.

3) Immunostimulant—The claim is that selenium given in amounts greater than ordinary nutritional requirements can significantly boost immune responses. Spallholz et al. (work reviewed in *Advances in Experimental Medicines and Biology*, 135:43, 1981) have demonstrated large increases in antibody production following administration of selenium in animal studies. Up to thirtyfold increases have been related to the administration of combination selenium/vitamin E. Soviet researchers have confirmed some of these findings. Desowitz and Barnewell (*Infection and Immunity*, 27:87, 1980) have reported that selenium added to the drinking water of mice in 2.5 ppm strongly potentiates immune response to malaria vaccine and reduces the fatality rate associated with subsequent re-exposure to malaria. Others have noted that selenium doubles the immune response to leptospirosis vaccine in calves.

Selenium deficiencies have been associated with marked impairment of the phagocytic cells that normally engulf foreign bodies. The lymphocytes of dogs have similarly shown impaired responses in the presence of selenium deficiency (*Federation Proceedings, Federation of the American Society for Experimen-*

tal Biology, 38:2139, 1979). Increased phagocytic activity is evidenced, on the other hand, in animals given supplemental selenium. Allograft rejection times have been shortened in mice and rabbits following selenium supplementation.

Selenium's immunostimulant mechanisms remain obscure. It has been suggested, however, that these mechanisms may be inferred, in part, from findings related to other antioxidants. High doses of vitamin E, for example, may have the ability to reduce the synthesis of immunosuppressive prostaglandins. Other research indicates that antioxidant nutrients help protect macrophages against the free radicals they generate to help destroy bacteria.

4) Protective against heart and circulatory diseases—Shamberger and group (*Proceedings of the Symposium on Selenium-Tellurium in the Environment*, Industrial Health Foundation, Pittsburgh, 1976, p. 253) have found epidemiological evidence that many forms of cardiovascular disease increase as selenium intake decreases. The so-called "stroke belt" of the U.S., an area encompassing part of Georgia and the Carolinas, is an area of very low selenium soil content. It has the highest stroke rate in the U.S. as well as a very high incidence of heart disease. In Finland, which also has very low selenium soil content and exceptionally high cardiovascular mortality, a long-term prospective study (*Lancet*, 2:175, 1982) of 11,000 Finns has revealed that blood levels of selenium of less than 45 micrograms per liter (a condition found in fully 30 percent of those studied) are associated with a death rate from acute coronary disease of nearly three times that of those with higher serum selenium. The rate of nonfatal heart attacks was also increased—to about twice that of those with higher blood levels of selenium. Keshan disease, a cardiomyopathy characterized by enlarged hearts and high death rates, has become endemic in areas of China that have particularly low selenium soil content. This disease has recently been reported (*Lancet*, Mar. 26, 1983, p. 685) to be responding to oral selenium supplementation.

A number of experimental studies suggest that selenium, especially in combination with vitamin E, may protect against tissue damage related to restricted blood flow or oxygen supply. In a double-blind study cited by Frost and Lish (*Annals of Pharmacology*, 18:259, 1975), 22 of 24 patients receiving 1 milligram of selenium and 200 IUs of vitamin E daily obtained significant relief from angina pain while only 5 of 24 patients on placebo were judged to have benefited similarly.

There is some evidence that selenium's potent antioxidant properties may inhibit some of the free-radical mechanisms that have been said to contribute to the sort of tissue damage discussed above. Its anticlotting effects appear related to its reported ability to inhibit blood platelet aggregation.

5) Capable of detoxifying heavy metals, various drugs, alcohol, cigarette smoke, peroxidized fats—Selenium's ability to detoxify a number of heavy metals, such as mercury and cadmium, has been widely reported (see Frost and Lish, cited above). The precise mechanism by which it does this is not known. In combining with the metals it may form inert, harmless selenides.

There is evidence selenium may detoxify peroxidized fats and thus inhibit their carcinogenicity. Several animal studies (see, for example, *American Journal of Veterinarian Research*, 39:997, 1978) have shown that selenium can significantly reduce the toxicity of the anticancer drug adriamycin without also reducing its antitumor activity. Some other studies, however, have failed to confirm this finding. Results are similarly mixed with respect to claims that selenium can protect against alcoholic liver disease. Claims that selenium confers protection against some forms of damage caused by cigarette smoking have not been adequately investigated.

6) Cosmetically beneficial to the skin—Claims that selenium increases the elasticity and "youthfulness" of the skin, removes "age spots" and so on have not been reliably investigated. Beneficial effects of selenium-sulfide shampoo to counteract dandruff and other exfoliative and seborrheic dermatitises have been reported.

7) Increases male potency and sex drive—Selenium is known to contribute significantly to sperm production and sperm motility. Restoration of fertility in some male diabetics has recently been reported following broad-spectrum antioxidant supplementation (including selenium). These reports, and those of increased sexual drive, remain purely anecdotal.

8) Anti-inflammatory and thus useful against arthritis and other autoimmune diseases—Injectable and oral selenium/vitamin E

preparations are used, with reported good results (see, for example, *Veterinarian Medicine and Small Animal Clinician*, 61:986, 1966), in veterinarian practice to relieve arthritic inflammation in dogs and other animals. Data on the use of selenium in human arthritis and other autoimmune diseases, however, are entirely lacking at this point.

RELATED TO NEGATIVE CLAIMS:

1) Highly toxic in even minute doses—The evidence cited above indicates that selenium can be tolerated in doses higher than was previously believed. See Recommendations: Suggested Intake below.

2) Mutagenic, i.e., capable of producing potentially harmful mutations in cells—Selenium in the form of sodium selenite has both mutagenic and antimutagenic effects under varying circumstances, but only at doses many times higher than would ordinarily be consumed. Equivalent doses of *organic* forms of selenium are not mutagenic. See Recommendations: Source/Form below.

3) Carcinogenic—See discussion of anticarcinogenic properties above. Most of the studies showing evidence of carcinogenicity are decades old. One epidemiological study in 1978, however, reported a higher colorectal-cancer mortality rate related to higher selenium levels in the drinking water. This finding has not been confirmed by other investigators. The National Research Council concluded in 1982 (*Diet, Nutrition and Cancer*, cited above) that "a critical review of the experimental conditions suggests that the earlier studies demonstrating carcinogenic or [cancer] promoting properties of selenium can be faulted on the basis of experimental design."

4) Cannot be effectively utilized by the body in supplement form—*Some* forms of selenium now on the market *cannot*, in fact, be effectively absorbed by the body. See Recommendations: Source/Form below.

5) Rendered useless by concurrent intake of vitamin C—See Recommendations: Source/Form below. Vitamin C taken at the

same time as sodium selenite can convert the selenium to a non-absorbable form.

IV. Recommendations

A) SUGGESTED INTAKE: The National Research Council lists the estimated safe and adequate dietary intake of selenium for adults and children seven years and older as 0.05 to 0.2 milligrams (50 to 200 *micrograms*) daily. That is, roughly, the estimated average for the American diet. Is it adequate? The evidence cited above would suggest that it may not be. Palmer et al. (*Journal of the American Dietetic Association*, 82:511, 1983) have recently shown that the upper limits proposed by the National Research Council are too low. Human doses in the range of 400 to 1,000 micrograms daily correspond to some of those dosages found to be anticarcinogenic or immunostimulant in animals, though this does not mean that smaller doses cannot also confer some of these same benefits. Some clinicians have reported using up to 1,000 micrograms of organic selenium daily in selected patients for prolonged periods without signs of toxicity.

There is sufficient reason to supplement diet with 100 to 200 micrograms of selenium daily. (Consult your physician before taking higher doses.) For children below seven years of age, supplemental intake should not exceed 100 micrograms daily. The form of the supplement is important; see below.

B) SOURCE/FORM: The best natural sources of selenium include broccoli, mushrooms, cabbage, celery, cucumbers, onions, radishes, brewer's yeast, grains, fish, organ meats. Remember, however, that even these foods may be very low in selenium, depending upon regional conditions. In general, soils in the eastern U.S. are more lacking in selenium than soils in the western U.S.

Selenium supplements can be obtained either in the form of inorganic sodium selenite or as organic selenium. Organic selenium is actually the major nutritional form of selenium, that is, the form that is present in the foods mentioned above. The organic forms available are usually derived from a special brewer's yeast enriched in selenium. There is evidence that the organic forms of selenium are preferable. Spallholz (unpublished data) has found that organic selenium yeast has a much lower potential for either toxicity or mutagenicity than the inorganic sodium selenite. Inorganic sodium selenite reacts with vitamin C in a way that decreases absorption of selenium. This is not true of organic selenium. Yang and co-workers (*American Journal of Clinical Nutrition*, 37:872, 1983) reported that long-term use of sodium selenite at 1 milligram per day or higher for prolonged periods has toxic effects. No toxicity has been reported with organic selenium in similar doses. In any case, it is not recommended that you take more than 200 *micrograms* of selenium daily.

C) TAKE WITH: Best if incorporated into a well-balanced vitamin/mineral "insurance" formula. (See Part Three for specific recommendations.) Because of widely reported synergistic effects, a daily 100 to 200-microgram dose of organic selenium may be accompanied by 100 to 400 IUs of vitamin E daily. Children under seven should take no more than 50 to 100 IUs of E with their selenium supplement.

D) CAUTIONARY NOTE: Don't take selenium with vitamin C if using the *inorganic* form of selenium, as explained above. Discontinue use of selenium if any signs of toxicity occur; these include garlic odor on breath and skin which persists, fragile or black fingernails, metallic taste, dizziness and nausea without other apparent cause. Toxicity is highly unlikely in the recommended dose/form. Be especially careful about high doses of this one.

Zinc

I. Overview

An increasing number of recent reports indicate zinc is necessary for optimal health. New findings suggest a very important role for zinc in maintaining the immune system and its ability to protect against disease. Recent evidence suggests that as we age we become increasingly prone to zinc deficiency (*American Journal of Clinical Nutrition*, 36:319, 1982). As a nutritional supplement, zinc is very much in the ascendancy.

More than one hundred enzymes (biologic catalysts) require

the trace metal zinc for their activity. Included are the enzymes that are involved in the production of nucleic acids DNA and RNA, the determinants of our biologic endowment. Zinc also plays a role in the structure and function of cell membranes. Signs of moderate to severe zinc deficiency include growth retardation, poor appetite, underfunctioning sex glands, mental lethargy, delayed wound healing, abnormalities of taste, smell and vision, skin changes and increased susceptibility to infection.

Although moderate to severe zinc deficiency is unlikely in developed countries, many groups in the population are at risk for marginal zinc deficiencies. Zinc deficiency is so common among hospital patients who are fed intravenously that hospitals are now adding zinc, along with other minerals, to the intravenous feeding solution.

Intriguing but still contradictory evidence related to zinc's possible role in cancer and cancer protection is slowly emerging. Zinc, the *preliminary* evidence suggests, may be useful in promoting healing of gastric ulcers and can be useful in treating *some* forms of male infertility and sexual impotence. Reports of zinc's usefulness in some forms of diabetes and in relieving some of the symptoms of rheumatoid arthritis are deserving of further study.

Adequate zinc intake is clearly necessary for optimal health and life-span.

II. Claims

POSITIVE:
1) Antioxidant; 2) boosts immunity; 3) prevents cancer; 4) required for maintenance of taste, smell and vision; 5) accelerates wound healing; 6) increases male potency and sex drive; 7) useful in the treatment and prevention of infertility; 8) prevents prostate problems; 9) useful in the treatment of acne; 10) prevents hair loss; 11) beneficial in diabetics; 12) anti-inflammatory and useful in the treatment of rheumatoid arthritis.

NEGATIVE:
1) Toxic.

III. Evidence

RELATED TO POSITIVE CLAIMS:

1) Antioxidant—Several lines of evidence suggest zinc to be an antioxidant, at least biologically. (See Part One for discussion of antioxidants and their anti-aging effects.) *Chemically*, one would expect zinc to be neither prooxidant nor antioxidant. However, biologically, zinc appears to be an antioxidant. Zinc is present in the structure of the enzyme copper-zinc superoxide dismutase, which plays a crucial role in the protection of cells against oxidant damage. The role of zinc in this enzyme, if any, has not yet been demonstrated. Zinc may protect against iron-induced free-radical damage. This is thought to be the case because zinc does influence other free-radical reactions. Iron, in its reduced form and interacting with oxygen, initiates free-radical peroxidation of polyunsaturated lipids, an activity that is definitely toxic to cells.

Studies with zinc-deficient chicks and animal red blood cells (*Nutrition Reviews*, 41:197, 1983) show that vitamin E can substitute for zinc in these situations to protect the cell membranes against peroxidation damage. Zinc functions as a membrane stabilizer in this capacity. Zinc is thought to bind to sulfhydryl groups in membranes and thus prevent their oxidation and maintain the membrane integrity by so doing. In addition, zinc is involved in the synthesis of the serum protein that carries vitamin A. Vitamin A is believed to be a singlet-oxygen quencher.

2) Boosts immunity—Here is another one of those rare instances where the often excessive or off-the-mark claims of the supplement marketplace have not yet caught up with the findings of medical science. There are research indications that adequate supplies of zinc are essential to the development and maintenance of a healthy immune system and that aging is associated with immune impairment that can sometimes be partially repaired with zinc supplementation.

It is clearly established, in fact, that zinc is essential for cell-mediated immunity (*Annual Review of Nutrition*, 2:151, 1982). The A46 mutant cattle of the Dutch Friesian type have a defect in the absorption of zinc leading to growth arrest, extreme susceptibility to infection and early death. They have impaired cellular immunity, but their humoral immunity is basically intact. The simple, successful treatment is zinc supplementation. Humans with the rare genetic disorder acrodermatitis enteropathica also have a problem with zinc absorption. Their easy susceptibility to infections leads to early death unless they are treated with zinc. The cellular limb of the immune system is mainly affected. The thymic wasting associated with protein-calorie malnutrition can be reversed with zinc supplements.

There are many groups in our population at increased risk of at least marginal zinc deficiency. We now know that the elderly, even the middle-to-upper-class elderly, may be getting insufficient zinc in their diets as manifested by decreased zinc levels (*Journal of Gerontology*, 26:358, 1971). The situation is even worse with the low-income elderly, who may be consuming less than 50 percent of the RDA for zinc. As people grow older there are significant alterations in their immune systems. These alterations form the basis for one of the theories of aging. Associated with aging is an increase in the production of antibodies against self, the so-called "autoimmune diseases," as well as an increased proneness to infections. Progressive zinc deficiency may play an important part in the gradual breakdown of the aging immune system.

A recent study (*American Journal of Medicine*, 70:1001, 1981) showed that zinc supplementation (in the amount of 220 milligrams of zinc sulfate twice a day for one month) increased the number of circulating T-lymphocytes, which fight infection, and improved antibody response in a group of healthy people over seventy years of age. There was no such improvement in a control group that received no supplementation.

These exciting findings justify further clinical trials to determine the effects of supplementary zinc on the immune system.

3) Prevents cancer—Contradictory findings abound with respect to this claim. Patients with esophageal cancer have been shown to have lower than normal levels of zinc in their blood (*Nutrition Reports International*, 15:635, 1977). Similar findings have been reported for those with bronchogenic cancer (*Journal of Clinical Pathology*, 21:363, 1968). Zinc levels are also significantly lower in men with cancer of the prostate than in men

with normal prostates (*Journal of Steroid Biochemistry*, 9:403, 1978). Zinc deficiency in rats is associated with an increased incidence of chemically induced esophageal cancer (*Journal of the National Cancer Institute*, 61:145, 1978). In other reports, adding zinc to hamster and rat diets inhibited chemically induced cancers (*Nature*, 231:447, 1971; *Journal of the National Cancer Institute*, 55:195, 1975).

So far, so good. But, unfortunately, there are also reports suggesting that tumor growth is slowed down in animals maintained on diets that are low in zinc (see, for example, *Journal of Parenteral and Enteral Nutrition*, 4:561, 1980). Schrauzer and co-workers (*Bioinorganic Chemistry*, 7:23, 1977, p. 35) found a direct correlation between estimated zinc intake and mortality from several different types of cancer, suggesting that zinc can *increase* some cancer risks.

How do we reconcile these differences? We have seen that zinc plays a pivotal role in immunity. A healthy immune system is undoubtedly important in protection against cancer, as evidenced, for example, by the occurrence of unusual malignancies in patients with so-called acquired immune deficiency syndrome (AIDS). The reports showing increased susceptibility to chemical carcinogenesis in zinc-deficient animals may relate to a problem of immune deficiency in these animals.

Another partial answer to this puzzle probably relates to zinc's interaction with other metals. When zinc antagonizes cadmium, the result may be *protection* against cancer. On the other hand, when zinc antagonizes selenium, the result may be an *increase* in cancer risk, since selenium is known to be protective against some cancers. Finally, it is not surprising that the rate of tumor growth is slower in zinc-deficient animals. Zinc is essential for nucleic-acid synthesis and thus is necessary for *all* growth, including malignant growth.

Since *marginal* zinc deficiency may be widespread, it is very important to clarify the issue of the role of zinc in the prevention of cancer through additional investigation.

4) Required for maintenance of taste, smell and vision—Abnormalities of taste, smell and vision are quite common as we age. Many older people do not have the same good appetite they had when they were young and they often blame this on food not tasting or smelling as good as it once did. The claim has been made that zinc can restore taste for these individuals.

Henkin and his associates (*Annals of Internal Medicine*, 99:227, 1983) showed that zinc deficiency clearly alters taste perception in animals and humans. Zinc deficiency can produce impaired taste acuity or unpleasant taste sensations. Altered taste sensitivity has been found to be related to disordered zinc metabolism in Crohn's disease, chronic renal failure, thermal burns, use of the drug penicillamine and in cystic fibrosis.

The clearest evidence that zinc supplementation can correct taste abnormalities is in uremic (kidney) patients on dialysis. But a study on the effect of zinc supplements on taste discrimination among the aged (*American Journal of Clinical Nutrition*, 31:633, 1978) found no significant improvement. It can be concluded that most age-related taste disorders are not due to zinc deficiency *alone*, although such a deficiency may certainly play a role.

Smell may also be impaired by zinc deficiency. Disorders of smell associated with some conditions of acquired zinc deficiency may be responsive to zinc supplementation. However, patients with disorders of smell for which the cause is unknown do not respond to zinc supplementation (*American Journal of the Medical Sciences*, 272:285, 1976).

There is no evidence that age-related disturbances in vision can be improved with zinc supplements.

5) Accelerates wound healing—Dramatic acceleration of surgical wound healing has been reported (*Annals of Surgery*, 165:432, 1967) among a group of patients who received zinc supplementation. Complete healing in 10 patients receiving 150 milligrams daily of elemental zinc in the form of zinc sulfate required forty-six days, while in a control group receiving no zinc supplementation, complete healing took eighty days. Another study (*Annals of Surgery*, 172:1048, 1970) failed to confirm this effect of zinc supplementation. It would seem that the value of zinc supplementation in wound healing is closely related to the zinc status of the individual. Enhanced wound healing is to be expected in zinc-deficient individuals following zinc therapy, since zinc is necessary for cellular repair. There is still some question, though, if supplemental zinc is useful in this respect in zinc-*sufficient* individuals. In any event, since zinc intake is barely adequate in many groups, it seems reasonable to give zinc supplements for optimal wound healing. To really settle the matter, however, more controlled studies will be required.

Frommer (*Medical Journal of Australia*, 2:793, 1975) reported that zinc-sufficient patients with gastric-ulcer disease who were given zinc supplements (150 milligrams of elemental zinc per day in the form of zinc sulfate) had an ulcer-healing rate three times that of patients treated with placebos. In addition, complete healing of ulcers occurred more frequently in the patients taking zinc than in the patients given placebos. Frommer's report warrants further study.

6) Increases male potency and sex drive—It is claimed that even marginal zinc deficiency can produce impotence. It is certain that moderate to severe deficiency produces regression of the male sex glands, the testes. Mild deficiency leads to low sperm count (*Nutrition Today*, Mar./Apr., 1981). Males with moderate to severe zinc deficiency exhibit decreased sexual interest as well as mental lethargy, emotional problems, poor appetite and all the other consequences of zinc deficiency. Antoniou and her associates (*Lancet*, 2:897, 1977), in their studies of sexually impotent males who were suffering from chronic kidney failure and who had low levels of zinc in their blood, reported a marked improvement in sexual potency in those patients who had zinc added to their hemodialysis solutions. This was accompanied by an increase in blood levels of the male sex hormone and in follicle-stimulating hormone. No such changes were observed in patients who got placebos instead of zinc.

Zinc and testosterone, the male sex hormone, are known to be closely interrelated, though the nature of this relationship remains unclear. The prostate gland is one of the organs richest in zinc. Prostatic zinc increases with puberty, and it is thought that testosterone is the main factor governing the zinc level of the prostate (*Investigative Urology*, 18:32, 1980). One of the functions of zinc may be to control testosterone metabolism at the cellular level. Zinc is thought to regulate the metabolism of testosterone in the prostate.

Hartoma and co-workers (*Lancet*, 2:1125, 1977) found that in males with mild zinc deficiency, zinc supplementation was accompanied by increased sperm count and plasma testosterone. It was not clear if potency was likewise affected. It appears that zinc supplementation is useful in counteracting male impotence only in the context of moderate to severe deficiency of this mineral. Many forms of male impotence have psychological bases and are otherwise unrelated to zinc. The effect of zinc on female sexual function is purely anecdotal.

7) Useful in the treatment and prevention of infertility—Zinc is known to be essential for sperm formation. Males who are moderately to severely zinc deficient may produce almost no sperm cells, while males who are mildly zinc deficient have reduced sperm counts. Zinc deficiency is also accompanied by a decreased testosterone level. The role of zinc in female infertility is unknown.

Of course, infertility also exists in men who are apparently zinc sufficient. Could zinc supplementation help *them?* Here I will be personal. My wife and I had been married for sixteen years before we had our first child. For at least ten years during that period we tried very hard to make a child. The problem seemed to be me. My sperm count was low, and the motility and morphology (ability to move and overall development) of the sperm cells were abnormal. I had been a cigarette smoker much of that time. I remembered that cadmium was present in cigarette paper. Cadmium is a zinc antagonist and could cause problems with sperm formation. I started taking 50 milligrams of zinc a day in the form of zinc gluconate. Within a few months my sperm count, as well as the morphology and motility of the cells, was normal. In no time our first child was conceived. Admittedly, this is anecdotal. However, cadmium exposure is very common via cigarette smoking and industrial exposure. Heavy exposure to cadmium, research suggests, may lead to softening of the bones, possibly to prostate cancer, renal disease, hypertension, anemia and lung disease. We're all exposed to cadmium. The average American accumulates 30 milligrams, mainly in the kidneys. The effects of mild exposure are unknown. I propose that mild cadmium exposure may lead to problems with sperm production because of its antagonism with zinc. Research of this issue is needed.

8) Prevents prostate problems—As discussed above, there is a great deal of zinc in the prostate. Enlargement of the prostate (benign prostatic hyperplasia) commonly occurs with aging. Supplementary zinc has been recommended for both the prevention and treatment of this condition. There is no evidence, however, that it does either. More research will have to be done

before any definite conclusions can be reached with respect to this claim.

9) Useful in the treatment of acne—Acne vulgaris is a chronic inflammation that primarily affects the adolescent age group. It is argued that adolescents develop an increased need for zinc that is not supplied by the diet and that the marginal zinc deficiency that results contributes to acne. There is no proof this is the case, though zinc therapy has been helpful in the treatment of acne in patients with *severe* zinc deficiency. Cunliffe (*British Journal of Dermatology*, 101:321, 1979) reported that oral zinc is as good as tetracycline for acne sufferers with severe zinc deficiency. Some others have failed to confirm this, however, so the evidence that oral zinc is helpful in the treatment of acne remains meager. More research is needed.

Topical zinc, on the other hand, does appear to be useful in treating acne, especially when it is combined with the antibiotic erythromycin (*Pediatric Clinics of North America*, 30:501, 1983). Topical zinc may act as an anti-inflammatory agent and help decrease production of the sebum that contributes to clogging the pores and causing acne.

10) Prevents hair loss—A few reports show that supplementary zinc restores hair growth in a few individuals with alopecia areata totalis (complete lack of body hair). There is no evidence that zinc restores hair to those suffering from typical male pattern baldness. And there is no evidence that supplementation with zinc will prevent hair loss.

11) Beneficial in diabetics—Insulin is the major hormone of sugar metabolism. Zinc appears to be involved with insulin at a few stages. Insulin is stored in the beta cells of the pancreas as a zinc crystal; zinc enhances the binding of insulin to liver cells and is involved with insulin in promoting the synthesis of lipids in fat cells. Rats that are deprived of zinc develop glucose intolerance (*Biological Trace Element Research*, 3:13, 1981).

Kinlaw and co-workers (*American Journal of Medicine*, 75:273, 1983) have recently reported that 25 percent of a group of diabetics who do not require insulin injections had depressed blood zinc levels as well as excessive zinc excretion in their urine. The authors suggest that these patients have problems absorbing zinc as well as overexcreting it in the urine. Why these patients malabsorb zinc is unclear.

Diabetics suffer from many complications such as poor wound healing and increased susceptibility to infections. Zinc plays an important role in both wound healing and in immune response. If it is true that a large percentage of diabetics are zinc deficient because of zinc malabsorption and hyperexcretion of zinc, then zinc supplementation would certainly be indicated in this group. Zinc supplementation could reduce diabetic complications. High-fiber diets are important in the management of diabetics, and this fact is relevant here because fiber *decreases* the body's ability to absorb zinc. This makes special consideration of zinc supplementation in diabetes an even more urgent matter. More research is needed.

12) Anti-inflammatory and useful in the treatment of rheumatoid arthritis—As indicated above, topical zinc may have anti-inflammatory properties and in that respect may be useful against acne. Chapil (*Medical Clinics of North America*, 60:799, 1976) has accumulated evidence in animal experiments that zinc supplementation results in the inhibition of several functions of some of the cells involved in immunity and prevents the release of histamine from mast cells. These actions should have anti-inflammatory effects, but more research will have to be done in order to determine the precise role of zinc.

Lower levels of serum zinc have been found in patients with rheumatoid arthritis than in normal individuals (*Journal of Chronic Diseases*, 23:527, 1971). Simkin (*Lancet*, 2:539, 1976) reported a trial of zinc supplementation in 24 patients with chronic rheumatoid arthritis of the sort that had not been helped by other treatments. In a double-blind study comparing zinc sulfate with a placebo, he found that the zinc-treated patients did better than the controls with regard to joint swelling, morning stiffness, walking time and the patients' own impressions of their overall disease activity. It is hypothesized that zinc is essential for the normal functioning of the joints and that local zinc deficiency is responsible to some extent for rheumatoid condition of joints. Zinc supplementation may lead to increased levels of zinc within the joints where the mineral's possible anti-inflammatory activity can impact directly upon the rheumatoid process.

There has been very little recent investigation of zinc's possible anti-inflammatory capabilities. Perhaps the interest in the nonsteroid anti-inflammatory drugs has crowded out any follow-up work on zinc in this area. This is too bad; zinc deserves further study to define the possible role it may play in rheumatoid arthritis, its treatment and prevention.

RELATED TO NEGATIVE CLAIMS:

1) Toxic—Zinc is thought to be relatively nontoxic (*Western Journal of Medicine*, 130:133, 1979). Some people have been taking up to 150 milligrams of elemental zinc each day for a few months (e.g., for rheumatoid arthritis, wound healing) with only occasional complaints of gastrointestinal problems, such as nausea, vomiting, diarrhea, epigastric distress and colic. However, recently some side effects have been observed in patients taking large doses of zinc over extended periods of time. Hopper and co-workers (*Journal of the American Medical Association*, 244:1960, 1980) reported that in young men large doses of zinc (150 milligrams of elemental zinc daily) depress high-density lipoprotein cholesterol levels. This is undesirable because high-density lipoprotein cholesterol is thought to protect against coronary heart disease. This study needs follow-up.

Zinc competes with copper for intestinal absorption; thus high doses of zinc may create a copper deficiency. Copper deficiency in rats causes an increase in low-density lipoprotein cholesterol, also bad because this form of cholesterol *increases* the risks of coronary heart disease, and a relative decrease in high-density lipoprotein cholesterol (*Nutrition Reports International*, 22:295, 1980). Klevay (*American Journal of Clinical Nutrition*, 28:764, 1975) believes that an elevated zinc/copper ratio, which could occur in the context of a patient taking large amounts of zinc, is an important risk factor for coronary heart disease. Porter and co-workers (*Lancet*, 2:774, 1977) report that a woman treated with zinc (150 milligrams of elemental zinc daily) for fourteen months developed a profound anemia due to copper deficiency. Thus, patients who need to take large doses of zinc, for medical reasons, should be given copper supplementation.

There are no reports of the long-term effects of low-dose supplementation with zinc. Many people take 30 to 50 milligrams of elemental zinc daily. Even in this dose range, however, it is advisable to include supplemental copper whenever zinc is taken.

IV. Recommendations

A) SUGGESTED INTAKE: The National Research Council's Recommended Daily Allowances (RDAs) for zinc are (expressed as elemental zinc): 15 milligrams for adults, 3 milligrams for infants less than six months old and 5 milligrams for infants between six months and one year, 10 milligrams for children from one year to ten years of age. To this, an additional 5 milligrams are recommended for pregnant women and 10 milligrams for those lactating (nursing infants). The optimal zinc intake for maximal longevity with minimal disease has not been defined.

There are many factors that make it difficult for us to be sure that we are getting enough zinc in our diets. Zinc content varies a great deal among different foods. And the amount of zinc that we absorb from these foods is influenced by many different things. The aged appear to be at particular risk of marginal zinc deficiency. They—and particularly those who eat mainly vegetarian diets—may be getting less than two-thirds, and in some cases less than one-half, the RDA. Our ability to absorb zinc decreases with age. High-fiber diets also diminish the amount of zinc we are able to absorb and utilize in our bodies. Athletes and dieters are at higher risk of zinc deficiency than most others, except for the aged and the vegetarians. Certain drugs (such as diuretics) and various disease states (such as diabetes and chronic alcoholism) lead to increased zinc excretion and thus to a need for increased zinc intake. Excessive sweating (as in the case of runners, athletes, etc.) can also cause significant zinc loss. There are compensatory mechanisms in the body that try to make up for these losses, but it is unclear if they are always adequate.

We can reasonably conclude that zinc intake may be barely adequate in many people, even in "healthy" and "well-fed" people. This inadequate or borderline-adequate intake may prove particularly troublesome in situations where increased zinc is required, e.g., the growing child, pregnancy, infection, convalescence, etc.

I believe that a zinc supplement is a prudent form of "insurance." I recommend between 15 to 30 milligrams daily for adults and 10 milligrams daily for children. Consult your physician before taking higher doses. It is noteworthy that many of the currently available children's and pregnant women's vitamin/mineral formulas do not contain zinc. Only recently has zinc been added to some children's cereals; this is fortunate in view of the fact that some children seem to eat almost nothing but cereals.

B) SOURCE/FORM: Dietary sources of zinc include whole-grain products, brewer's yeast, wheat bran and germ; seafoods and animal meats are, in general, much better sources of bioavailable (easily absorbed) zinc than are vegetables. There are several zinc supplements on the market: zinc sulfate, zinc acetate, zinc gluconate, zinc citrate and amino chelates of zinc. There is some evidence that the protein breakdown products (amino acids and their derivatives) naturally facilitate the absorption of zinc (*Journal of Nutrition*, 113:1346, 1983). *Any* of the above forms of zinc are acceptable since they will all be converted to the appropriate natural form in the body. The amount of elemental zinc available in each preparation varies depending on the degree of hydration of the zinc complex. The amount of elemental zinc is commonly listed on the product label as the "zinc equivalent."

C) TAKE WITH: Best if incorporated into a well-balanced vitamin/mineral formula. (See Part Three for further recommendations.) Specifically, I suggest that a daily 15-to-30-milligram dose of zinc be accompanied by 2–3 milligrams of copper and 200 micrograms of selenium for the reasons already discussed. The ratio of zinc to copper should be about 10:1 (milligram to milligram). Therefore, if a physician recommends higher intakes of zinc, the copper dose can be adjusted using this ratio.

D) CAUTIONARY NOTE: Toxicity at the recommended dose is highly unlikely. See discussion under Related to Negative Claims with respect to higher doses.

six

AMINO ACIDS

Amino acids have only recently been marketed widely as individual food supplements. In order to make sense of these substances it is important to define some terms. In principle, an amino acid is any compound that contains an amino group and an acidic function. This definition includes a wide variety of substances, many of which have no known biological function. When biologists talk about amino acids, they usually mean the twenty amino acids that are necessary for the synthesis of proteins. Proteins are large molecules that are crucial to life; they are involved in the formation of living structure and they catalyze the chemical reactions necessary for the maintenance of life.

The twenty amino acids that form the building blocks of all proteins are alanine, arginine, asparagine, aspartic acid, cysteine, glutamic acid, glutamine, glycine, histidine, isoleucine, leucine, lysine, methionine, phenylalanine, proline, serine, threonine, tryptophan, tyrosine, and valine. There are other amino acids found in our bodies such as taurine and ornithine, but these amino acids are not involved in the synthesis of proteins.

In addition to participating in the synthesis of proteins, amino acids are involved in other important biological processes such as the formation of the brain neurotransmitters. There are some recent studies which suggest that certain amino acids may play important roles in enhancing the immune system and protecting against cancer.

The twenty amino acids involved in protein biosynthesis are divided into two broad groups—essential and nonessential. Healthy human adults require dietary intake of eight of these amino acids to maintain good health: phenylalanine, valine, threonine, tryptophan, isoleucine, methionine, lysine and leucine. The remaining twelve—the nonessential amino acids— can be made by the body from other substances. Healthy children require, in addition to the eight amino acids listed above, histidine and arginine. Situations exist in which nonessential amino acids become essential. For example, a physically traumatized adult requires arginine for optimal repair processes to occur.

Some promising pharmacological applications are emerging for amino-acid supplements, especially in the realm of behavioral modification.

In the analyses that follow, emphasis is on those amino acids for which anti-aging claims have been made, especially L-arginine and L-cysteine.

L-arginine (With a Note on Ornithine)

I. Overview

L-arginine is currently a hot item in the food-supplement marketplace. Its growing appeal has been fueled by claims that it niftily manages to burn fat while building muscle. Arginine does, in fact, have a definite stimulating effect on human growth hormone, which, in turn, has a number of remarkable properties. This does not mean that the time has come to take large quantities of arginine (such a practice could prove risky, especially without medical supervision), but preliminary research results suggest that arginine may have an important future as a pharmacologic agent if not as a routine food supplement.

Arginine's sudden surge in popularity in the health-food market is particularly interesting in view of the fact that it has long been regarded as something of a villain in that same marketplace for its purported role in promoting the herpes virus (see Related to Negative Claims below).

II. Claims

POSITIVE:
1) Burns fat and builds muscle; 2) speeds wound healing; 3) stimulates the immune system; 4) inhibits cancer; 5) increases sexual fertility in males.

NEGATIVE:
1) Excessive intake may cause bone and skin disorders; 2) causes nausea and diarrhea; 3) promotes herpes.

III. Evidence

RELATED TO POSITIVE CLAIMS:

1) Burns fat and builds muscle—Dieters, athletes, body-builders and others are using arginine increasingly for its reputed ability to rid the body of fat and imbue it with muscle. The claim is that arginine stimulates the pituitary gland in the brain in such a way that increased amounts of growth hormone (GH) are released into the bloodstream. GH, in turn, is said to help burn fat and build muscle. It has, in fact, been demonstrated (*Current Medical Research and Opinion*, 7:475, 1981) that oral intake of arginine in combination with lysine caused the release of biologically active quantities of GH. It is interesting to note, however, that without the additional amino acid lysine, arginine did not produce a significant increase in GH—interesting because the popular claims for arginine have not made any reference to lysine. But, then, most of those claims have been based upon findings in animals other than man. Further study will be

required to determine to what extent oral arginine alone can stimulate GH in humans. In the study cited above, 1,200 milligrams of lysine were given with 1,200 milligrams of arginine. The study, however, did not demonstrate either a "fat burning" or a "muscle building" effect; that wasn't part of its design. To date, no controlled experiments in humans have been conducted to see whether arginine really can trim body fat and/or build muscle. Such experiments are needed. Given what we know about GH it is not unreasonable to expect that arginine, if its stimulating effects on GH are consistent and potent, could do these things—though to what extent and at what possible risk also remain to be elucidated.

2) Speeds wound healing—Seifter and co-workers (*Surgery*, Aug. 1978, p. 224) reported that arginine supplements significantly accelerated wound healing in rats while simultaneously retarding the weight loss that usually accompanies physical trauma. These positive effects were attributed in part to arginine's ability to stimulate secretion of growth hormone, which, it is speculated, may favorably influence the synthesis of those proteins that contribute to the reparative process. These researchers concluded that "arginine plays an important role in post-injury phenomena, e.g., weight changes, nitrogen balance, and wound healing." And they suggested that any patients hospitalized for various injuries might benefit from increased arginine (via intravenous feeding). This promising work needs to be expanded and controlled inquiry initiated into the possible effects of arginine on human injury.

3) Stimulates the immune system—Barbul and colleagues (*Journal of Parenteral and Enteral Nutrition*, 4:446, 1980) demonstrated that arginine supplementation stimulates the thymus gland and various thymic processes associated with enhanced immunity. Mice given arginine supplements exhibited thymic growth, increased thymic lymphocytes (cells crucial to immunity) and more highly active lymphocytes. Again, these potentially beneficial effects were attributed to arginine's ability to stimulate growth hormone, which, in turn, stimulates thymic activity. These researchers concluded that arginine can enhance immune defense systems; extrapolating from the findings in mice they suggested that similar effects might be seen in humans and that "severely injured or ill patients" might benefit

from arginine supplementation in excess of those amounts normally considered adequate. It is interesting to note that the positive effects seen in this study were observed in mice that were not deficient, by accepted standards, in arginine. This suggests, but does not prove, that intake of arginine in excess of nutritional needs (the amount of which has not been settled) may be beneficial in some cases.

It is never entirely safe, however, to extrapolate from mouse to man, as these researchers recognized. Thus, they conducted a preliminary study (*Surgery*, Aug. 1981, p. 244) of the effects of arginine on the immune response of healthy human volunteers, all of whom received (orally) 30 grams of arginine daily for a week. Test-tube studies of the lymphocytes of these arginine-augmented volunteers revealed dramatically enhanced activity, which, "translated to the living host," the researchers stated, suggests "a greater ability of lymphocytes to respond to antigenic challenges," that is, to infections. These promising preliminary findings in healthy subjects (a required first step) "encourages us," these researchers concluded, "to pursue its applications in patients with immunosuppression secondary to injury, surgical trauma, malnutrition and sepsis. . . . We believe that supplemental arginine may provide a safe, non-toxic, nutritional means of boosting the immune response of these patients and we are in the process of studying this application."

There is some further, still very preliminary evidence (Barbul, personal communication) that arginine selectively boosts the activity of the so-called "helper" lymphocytes—without, at the same time, also boosting the activity of the "suppressor" lymphocytes. This is a favorable finding—if confirmed—because various serious disorders, including AIDS (acquired immune deficiency syndrome), are characterized by heightened suppressor/diminished helper lymphocyte activity.

This is not to say that arginine will prove useful against such diseases as AIDS (far more study will be required before its impact can be assessed); nor should consumers overlook the fact that when these researchers call arginine, in the huge doses used, "safe," they are talking about its use for short periods of time in severely ill patients under a doctor's continual care and observation. It most definitely has not been established that it is safe for people to routinely take large doses of arginine. Nor should the consumer forget that to date there has been no reason established for normal people to take large doses of arginine.

Further, as Barbul and his co-workers acknowledge, only further studies will determine for sure whether the immune-stimulating effects observed to date are truly beneficial and/or lasting. This is exciting work that bears watching; we'll provide further information in future editions of this book.

4) Inhibits cancer—Arginine supplementation has been shown to inhibit the growth of various tumors in laboratory animals. Rettura and co-workers (*Journal of Parenteral and Enteral Medicine*, 3:409, 1979) correlated the thymus-stimulating effects (see discussion above of immune-enhancing effects) of arginine with a significant antitumor effect in a cancer caused by a virus. Here again, then, arginine's ability to increase growth-hormone secretion seems to be the key. Milner and Stepanovich (*Journal of Nutrition*, 109:489, 1979) have also reported an arginine-related antitumor effect in mice. "Arginine," they conclude, "represents a nutrient required for optimum growth of normal tissue, yet may be capable of retarding tumor development." Mechanisms by which arginine may do this, beyond its effect on the immune system, have not been elucidated, though it does appear that there are additional mechanisms. Again, more work is needed to follow up on this exciting early finding.

5) Increases sexual fertility in males—Shettles reported some years ago (*Fertility and Sterility*, 11:88, 1960) that arginine is essential in man and many lower animals for normal sperm production. More recently, others (*Journal of Urology*, 110:311, 1973) reported successfully treating a number of men suffering from low sperm count with arginine. Many of these men had previously been treated with a wide selection of vitamins, hormones and antibiotics without improvement in their sperm counts. More than 80 percent of the men given 4 grams of oral arginine daily enjoyed moderate to marked increases in sperm count and motility. At the time the report was written twenty-eight pregnancies had resulted and more were expected.

RELATED TO NEGATIVE CLAIMS:

1) Excessive intake may cause bone and skin disorders—This fear has been voiced with respect, particularly, to the ingestion of large doses of supplemental arginine by nonadults in whom long-bone growth is not yet complete. There is no absolute

proof that large doses of arginine will result in bone deformities in this group, but given arginine's ability to affect growth hormone (and sometimes in unpredictable ways and varying from one individual to the next), nonadults are strongly advised not to take arginine supplements. There have also been anecdotal reports of abnormal growth following prolonged ingestion of large amounts of arginine.

2) Causes nausea and diarrhea—Very large doses of arginine have produced these side effects in a matter of a few days in some individuals. These side effects disappear soon after arginine is discontinued or intake is moderated.

3) Promotes herpes—The relative intake of arginine and lysine has been reported (see discussion of lysine later in this chapter) to promote the activity of some of the herpes viruses. This association has not yet been proved, although there is some preliminary, unconfirmed evidence that high arginine/low lysine intake may favor herpes growth. This hypothesis needs further investigation.

IV. Recommendations

A) SUGGESTED INTAKE: Optimal intake is unknown. At this time I do not recommend taking arginine supplements in any quantity except under medical supervision. If you have a problem that you believe might be benefited by arginine supplements, discuss the matter with a physician, calling attention to data cited in this book.

B) SOURCE/FORM: Natural sources of arginine include raw cereals, chocolate, various nuts.

C) CAUTIONARY NOTE: Remember that the preliminary, favorable effects reported in the literature were achieved with extremely high doses that may not be safe in humans for prolonged periods of time. Young people (all nonadults) whose long-bone growth is not yet complete should not take arginine supplements at all as bone deformities are a possibility in this group (see Evidence: Related to Negative Claims above).

NOTE ON ORNITHINE—Ornithine is another amino acid you are likely to find heavily touted in the health-food literature. Ornithine is readily available in most vitamin stores. It is linked here to arginine because it too has been shown to be capable of increasing the body's secretion of growth hormone (though the doses required to do this are, again, very large and potentially quite risky). Less research has been done on ornithine, but it too has been shown to stimulate the thymus gland of laboratory animals, possibly enhancing immune response in the process (*Federation Proceedings, Federation of the American Society for Experimental Biology*, 37:264, 1978). In addition, ornithine has exhibited liver-regenerating effects in animals (*Biochimica et Biophysica Acta*, 190:193, 1969). Foods rich in ornithine include meats and dairy products.

L-cysteine
(And Glutathione)

I. Overview

Cysteine is one of the amino acids that contain sulfur in a form that is said to inactivate free radicals and thus protect and preserve cells. Claims are made that various sulfur-containing antioxidants can extend life-span and protect against various toxic substances. (Methionine and taurine, discussed later in this chapter, are other sulfur-containing amino acids.) Cysteine is a precursor of glutathione, a tripeptide, it is claimed, that can protect the body against various pollutants.

II. Claims

POSITIVE:
1) Extends life-span; 2) protects against toxins and pollutants, including some found in cigarette smoke and alcohol; 3) combats arthritis.

NEGATIVE:
1) Contributes to kidney stones; 2) dangerous for diabetics; 3) toxic.

III. Evidence

RELATED TO POSITIVE CLAIMS:

1) Extends life-span—Oeriu and Vachitsu (*Journal of Gerontology*, 20:417, 1965) injected guinea pigs and mice with cysteine every other day for more than a month. They reported significantly increased survival times in these animals. Harmon (*Revue Francaise Gerontology*, 9:125, 1963) similarly noted marked increases in survival time among cysteine-supplemented mice. Tas et al. have noted (*Mechanisms of Ageing and Development*, 12:65, 1980) an age-related decrease in those sulfur-containing substances that are hypothesized to protect against aging through antioxidant and other influences. Weitzman and Stossel (*Immunology*, 128:2770, 1982) have suggested that cysteine may participate in some forms of DNA repair, another mechanism that, theoretically, could help inhibit aging. Cysteine is an established antioxidant, but its anti-aging effects remain to be demonstrated in man. Even the animal work, though intriguing, is far from conclusive. More work needs to be done.

2) Protects against toxins and pollutants, including some found in cigarette smoke and alcohol—Aldehydes, toxic products of some fats, alcohol, smoke, smog, etc., are said to be partially neutralized by cysteine. One group (*Federation Proceedings, Federation of the American Society for Experimental Biology*, Abstract No. 172, Mar. 1974, p. 233) reported that large doses of alcohol-derived acetaldehyde killed 90 percent of the rats to which it was given. Another group of rats were first given quantities of vitamins C and B_1, along with cysteine, then were exposed to the same doses of acetaldehyde that had proved fatal in most of the other group of rats. *None* of the vitamin/cysteine-augmented rats died. There have been other reports that cysteine can protect against other potentially toxic substances. Cysteine is a precursor of glutathione, a tripeptide (made from three amino acids) which has been reported to eliminate certain toxic chemicals by binding to them and thus rendering them harmless. Edes and collaborators (*Proceedings of the Society for Experimental Biology and Medicine*, 162:71, 1979) report that rats fed methionine- and cysteine-deficient diets have lower lev-

els of enzymes that are protective against carcinogens. Further research is indicated.

3) Combats arthritis—British research (reported upon in *Medical World News*, Oct. 7, 1978) indicated that cysteine given in conjunction with pantothenic acid (see discussion of pantothenic acid and royal jelly elsewhere in this book) had positive effects on patients suffering from osteoarthritis and rheumatoid arthritis. At this point, however, there is insufficient evidence to support the claim that cysteine can alleviate the symptoms of any form of arthritis, though the preliminary British study deserves follow-up.

RELATED TO NEGATIVE CLAIMS:

1) Contributes to kidney stones—There have been no studies showing that cysteine supplementation will result in kidney stones, though the fear that it might is not entirely without foundation. Even most of the cysteine enthusiasts caution people on this score, urging that vitamin C be taken along with cysteine to help prevent it from converting to cystine, a close relative, which could, in fact, cause bladder and/or kidney stones. The recommended combination is two to three times as much vitamin C as cysteine.

2) Dangerous for diabetics—There is some evidence that cysteine may interfere with insulin; diabetics are therefore advised not to use cysteine supplements without consulting their physicians.

3) Toxic—There are anecdotal reports that cysteine can increase the toxicity of monosodium glutamate in individuals who suffer from the so-called "Chinese restaurant syndrome," a set of symptoms, including headache, burning sensations, and sometimes dizziness and disorientation, that follows the ingestion of monosodium-glutamate-laced foods.

IV. Recommendations

A) SUGGESTED INTAKE: Optimal intake is unknown. I do not recommend taking cysteine supplements except under a doctor's supervision. If you have problems that you believe might be helped by cysteine supplementation, consult your physician, calling attention to data cited above.

B) SOURCE/FORM: Good dietary sources of cysteine include eggs, meat, dairy products and some cereals.

C) TAKE WITH: If you do take cysteine supplements (not recommended), take with vitamin C (two to three times as much vitamin C as cysteine, milligram to milligram) as a precaution against kidney- and/or bladder-stone formation.

D) CAUTIONARY NOTE: Diabetics should not take cysteine supplements unless directed to do so by a physician who is aware of the diabetes. (Also see information related to kidney stones and "Chinese restaurant syndrome" under Evidence: Related to Negative Claims above.)

Other Amino Acids of Current Interest

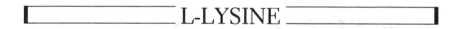

L-LYSINE

Lysine is enjoying brisk sales these days owing to widely publicized claims that it is effective against some of the sexually transmissible herpes viruses that cause painful lesions in the oral and genital areas. Lysine serves several vital functions in the body, but so far no significant claims have been made for it as a life extender. The herpes data, meanwhile, remain inconclusive at best. Most of the claims for lysine are based on the studies of Kagan (*Lancet*, 1:37, 1974) and Kagan and co-workers (*Dermatologica*, 156:257, 1978). These studies claimed to find lysine of benefit in the treatment of herpes. Because they hypothesized that arginine promotes herpes activity, while lysine inhibits it, subjects were instructed to cut back on arginine-rich foods, in addition to taking lysine supplements (up to a gram a day during active outbreak of the virus). The first of these studies was very small and was uncontrolled. The second study involved more patients but was similarly without placebos or control patients for comparison. Except in a few cases there was no objective confirmation (via tissue culture) of herpes. The reported benefits (which have been enormously distorted by some of the lysine promoters and enthusiasts) were largely subjective: there *seemed* to be fewer outbreaks of active herpes and milder symptoms once outbreaks did occur. The researchers themselves acknowledged the need for better controlled studies.

A better study—the results of which have been carefully ignored by the "lysine lobby"—was forthcoming later in 1978, conducted by Danish scientists. This well-designed double-blind, placebo-controlled trial of lysine (*Lancet*, Oct. 28, 1978, p. 942) failed to confirm Kagan and co-workers. Of 104 patients participating, 53 received a gram of lysine a day while the 51 control patients received placebos. There was no difference in herpes recurrence rates or healing times. The researchers held out some hope, however, that future investigations with larger doses of lysine might yet reveal some preventive property. For now, such a property remains speculative.

There are anecdotal reports that larger doses of lysine do inhibit herpes, but there are also anecdotal reports that such doses are ineffective and even some reports that daily ingestion for preventive purposes predisposes to more frequent but less severe outbreaks. Anecdotal evidence is rarely reliable. At present there is no genuine scientific support for the claim that lysine inhibits herpes.

Dietary sources of lysine include red meats, milk, potatoes.

☐ METHIONINE AND TAURINE ☐

These are both sulfur-containing amino acids (see discussion of same under the analysis of cysteine, earlier in this chapter). There are unproved claims that methionine, which can be found in eggs, milk, liver, fish and many other foods, has therapeutic lipotropic activities similar to those of choline (see discussion of choline later in this book) which help eliminate fatty substances that might otherwise clog the arteries. Little useful research has been done on the possible therapeutic effects of methionine supplementation in humans. There is one study (*Biochemical and Biophysical Research Communications*, 61:525, 1974) that indirectly suggests that methionine is destroyed by excessive use of alcohol. But, in any event, there is no doubt that methionine is very important in numerous processes in man. It appears likely, moreover, that both cysteine (see discussion earlier) and taurine, two other important amino acids, depend in part upon adequate levels of methionine for their biosynthesis in the body.

Hayes and Sturman note, in an excellent review of the relevant literature (*Annual Review of Nutrition*, 1:401, 1981), that "taurine is rapidly emerging as one of the more interesting and ubiquitous of the amino acids." There is increasing evidence that taurine is an important regulator of various nerve and muscle systems and that it may be essential for proper growth. Mammalian species apparently differ to some extent in their relative abilities to biosynthesize (produce in their own bodies) taurine; most seem to require at least some in their diets. Human work is largely lacking, but cats have been shown (*Journal of Nutrition*, 108:1462, 1978) to suffer a tenfold reduction in tissue taurine levels a few months after having been placed on taurine-deficient diets. Some taurine is synthesized from methionine and cysteine, but eventually these sources prove inadequate and retinal degeneration is one of the consequences. (Very large quantities of taurine are found in the retina of the eye of many mammals.) Retarded growth has been noted in young monkeys (*Journal of Nutrition*, 110:119, 1980) fed taurine-free diets. More study will be required before any conclusions can be drawn about possible taurine deficiencies in man and the consequences thereof.

Those who are considering taurine supplements—and some are on the market—are advised that numerous studies (see Hayes and Sturman cited above) have shown that taurine has a *depressant* effect on the central nervous system and, according to these review authors, "may even have adverse effects on inhibitory or short-term labile memory functions." It is the nerve-depressant aspect of taurine that has attracted the interest of those concerned with epilepsy, which involves a state of neural *over*excitation. Taurine seems to inhibit and modulate various of the neurotransmitters, the chemical messengers of the brain. Barbeau and colleagues were the first (*Archives of Neurology*,

30:52, 1974; *Life Sciences*, 17:669, 1975) to report on the benefits of oral taurine in the treatment of human epilepsy. "We can confidently conclude at this time that taurine does exert definite, albeit mild, anticonvulsant activity in human epilepsy," these researchers concluded. Studies are ongoing to see whether taurine may be more useful in some instances than the standard anticonvulsants.

For now, supplementation with either taurine or methionine appears ill-advised, though these substances may be useful in certain individuals, when prescribed by physicians. These amino acids are present in meats and animal products but not in plant products.

⎡PHENYLALANINE AND TYROSINE⎤

Claims for the amino acids phenylalanine and tyrosine, both now widely available in supplement form, are sweeping. Unfortunately, these claims are not generally accompanied by the appropriate cautions. There are some serious potential health hazards associated with the use of these substances in supplement form that are discussed below. Both phenylalanine and tyrosine are involved in biochemical processes related to the synthesis of various neurotransmitters, principally dopamine and epinephrine. The popular claims are that these substances have neurological excitatory effects that dispel depression, improve memory, diminish pain, increase mental alertness and even promote "sexual interest." They are also supposed to release hormones that suppress appetite.

Rasmussen and co-workers (*Journal of Clinical Endocrinology and Metabolism*, 57:760, 1983) have shown that oral tyrosine can induce significant short-term increases in blood levels of norepinephrine, dopamine and epinephrine. Glaeser and co-workers (*Life Sciences*, 25:265, 1979) have produced similar results. Gelenberg and colleagues (*American Journal of Psychiatry*, 137:522, 1980) tested tyrosine on one depressed patient and reported favorable results. "Symptoms of depression decreased dramatically during tyrosine administration and recurred when placebo was substituted," these researchers noted, adding that "if tyrosine is demonstrated to be effective (in extensive further testing) and if it actually has few unwanted effects, it might become an attractive alternative to the antidepressants currently available." Goldberg (*Lancet*, 2:364, 1980) treated two long-depressed patients who had failed to respond to standard antidepressants and to electroconvulsive "shock" treatments. Goldberg reported improvement in both patients. Obviously, far more rigorous tests will have to be carried out before the claimed benefits of tyrosine and phenylalanine are supported or refuted.

In the meantime, the consumer is advised to avoid adding these substances to the diet in the form of supplements. There is experimental evidence (see review of Wurtman and group, *Pharmacological Reviews*, 32:315, 1981) that tyrosine can both lower and elevate blood pressure under different circumstances. There is evidence that phenylalanine supplements can also elevate blood pressure in some individuals. Persons taking antidepressant drugs containing monoamine oxidase inhibitors should, in particular, avoid both tyrosine and phenylalanine as the combination could dangerously elevate blood pressure. There have also been anecdotal reports that tyrosine supplements can trigger migraine headaches in those prone to them. Migraine patients, as a matter of fact, are sometimes counseled to avoid foods rich in tyrosine, such as cheese, bananas, beer, wine, avocado, pickled herring. Persons suffering from PKU (phenylketonuria), the inherited inability to metabolize phenylalanine, should, of course, avoid phenylalanine supplements and should adhere to diets low in this amino acid, as outlined by their doctors. Pigmented malignant melanoma, a particularly deadly form of skin cancer, it should also be noted, seems to be at least partially dependent upon tyrosine and phenylalanine for rapid growth.

There is no convincing evidence that either tyrosine or phenylalanine can stimulate or sustain sexual interest or arousal, improve or protect memory, or contribute to weight loss. These substances may have a significant future in the treatment of some forms of depression; if so, however, they will require medical supervision to guard against useless or dangerous misapplication and potentially hazardous side effects. There is some preliminary evidence (*Pain*, 8:231, 1980) that phenylalanine in combination with electroacupuncture is a more effective analgesic than electroacupuncture alone, but this finding too requires follow-up and confirmation.

⎯⎯⎯⎯⎯ TRYPTOPHAN ⎯⎯⎯⎯⎯

Tryptophan was one of the first of the individual amino acids to be marketed, primarily as a "natural sleep aid." Tryptophan is involved in the biosynthesis of a neurotransmitter called serotonin. Serotonin may be an inducer of certain stages of sleep, though its activity in this respect is not yet well understood. Wurtman has reported (*Lancet*, May 21, 1983, p. 1145) that healthy young men given a single dose of tryptophan in the morning "self-reported fatigue/inertia and reduced vigor/activity." Claims that tryptophan is an effective antidepressant have not been substantiated (*Pharmacological Reviews*, 32:315, 1981). Evidence related to the claim that tryptophan can suppress appetite is inconclusive. There is some preliminary evidence (*Hospital Practice*, July 1983, p. 100) that tryptophan may be able to decrease sensitivity to moderate but not severe pain. Research is ongoing with respect to possible roles of tryptophan in the treatment of mania and aggressive behavior; there is no conclusive evidence at this point that it is useful in either condition. More research is needed before any conclusions can be drawn even with respect to the principal claim made for tryptophan— that it is a safe and effective sleep aid. Certainly, given the serious side effects of many of the standard sleep medications, such research should be carried out. For the present, however, no one should assume that self-dosing with tryptophan is either beneficial or safe. Those who insist upon using tryptophan supplements should be aware that an association has been noted between high intake of tryptophan and cancer of the bladder in vitamin-B_6-deficient experimental animals (*Cancer Research*, 39:1207, 1979).

seven

NUCLEIC ACIDS AND DERIVATIVES

Some of the most important biomedical discoveries of all time were made during this century. They concern substances we call the nucleic acids. These are large biological molecules within which are encoded the genetic instructions that determine biological specificity, that is, whether we will be a bacterium, a cat, a human being or any number of other life forms. Nucleic-acid genetic material also helps determine what color and size we will be and even, to a certain extent, whether we will have a sweet or a sour disposition, an analytical or a creative frame of mind.

There are essentially two major categories of nucleic acids: deoxyribonucleic acid, or DNA, and ribonucleic acid, or RNA. The information that these acids impart depends upon the arrangement—the sequence—of molecules called the purine and pyrimidine bases. The bases that combine in various sequences to make up the "messages" of DNA are called adenine, guanine, thymine and cytosine. Adenine, guanine and cytosine are also found in RNA, but thymine is replaced by uracil. These individual bases are strung together along a backbone comprised of phosphate and a sugar called deoxyribose in the case of DNA and ribose in the case of RNA.

The genetic messages of "instructions" contained within DNA are transferred to RNA by a process known as "transcription." Once information is transferred or "transcribed" from DNA to RNA it is utilized to "build" biological matter by causing the twenty amino acids to line up in the proper sequences required to make protein. This process is called "translation." The formation of life thus depends upon the proper translation of the original genetic code contained in the DNA. The continuity of the DNA code is ensured by repair processes and by DNA replication. Cellular aging has been attributed to errors that occur during DNA repair, DNA replication, the synthesis of RNA (transcription) and the synthesis of proteins (translation).

It is not difficult to understand, then, why nucleic acids and various nucleic derivatives have become staples in the food-supplement supermarket. The makers of cosmetics too have been quick to incorporate RNA, DNA and derivatives into hair and skin products. The idea is that as we age, our DNA/RNA become depleted or, in any event, are prone to increasing "error." Thus, it is argued, we must "replace" our lost or ineffective nucleic acids with supplemental forms. This is, in a sense, an offshoot of "cellular therapy," where oral and injected preparations of young cells—from various tissues and organs— were given to replace "worn-out" tissues and organs in aging bodies.

The physician who is mainly responsible for the popularity of dietary and cosmetic nucleic acids is the late Dr. Benjamin S. Frank, who believed that *dietary* nucleic acids were essential for optimal health. His ideas were not widely accepted, however, because his results were largely anecdotal. Oral supplementation, moreover, doesn't make sense; these supplements are destroyed in the gut before they can get to target tissues. The whole concept of "cellular therapy" is naïve. We probably *do* experience breakdowns and shortages in nucleic acids and their machinery as we age, but oral supplementation is not going to do us any good. There is some evidence that synthetic *injected* preparations may have some pharmacological effects (discussed below), but these are not really related to the claims made in the popular literature. Perhaps one day we *will* be able to dramatically retard aging via nucleic-acid manipulation, but that will require sophisticated gene surgery—something that is still far in the future.

DNA and RNA

The popular claim is that nucleic-acid supplements retard the aging process, specifically that they improve memory, inhibit degenerative diseases and stimulate weakened immune systems. It is further claimed that as we age, our ability to synthesize DNA and RNA dramatically diminishes, making supplementation necessary. This has never been scientifically established in humans, however, and the animal data are contradictory and inconclusive (see review in *Geriatrics*, Oct. 1977, p. 130).

Frank (mentioned above) claimed (*Nucleic Acid and Anti-Oxidant Therapy of Aging and Degeneration*, Rainstone Publishing, New York, 1977) that animals supplemented with nucleic acids, various nucleic-acid components and precursors, amino acids, B vitamins and so on exhibited increased vigor, endurance and survival. He also noted a reduction of spontaneous mammary tumors in mice. In humans, Frank reported numerous therapeutic effects of nucleic-acid therapy, including improved cardiac function, improved liver function, enhanced mental acuity, and benefit in diabetes, glaucoma, nerve disorders, atherosclerosis and emphysema. He also reported that nucleic-acid therapy could improve the quality of skin, giving it a more youthful appearance. Unfortunately, Frank did not provide scientifically acceptable documentation for most of his findings. His studies were small and lacked controls; his conclusions were largely subjective.

Many years ago, Newman and Grossman (*American Journal of Physiology*, 164:251, 1951) conducted experiments suggesting that nucleic-acid supplements can speed the rate of liver regeneration in rats. Later, Odens (*Journal of the American Geriatrics Society*, 21:450, 1973) reported that rats injected weekly with DNA and RNA lived twice as long as control rats that did not receive these substances. Though intriguing, this latter study has not been accorded much attention, owing to the small number (five) of rats injected with RNA/DNA. This experiment bears repeating.

In another animal study (*Cancer Research*, 31:4, 1971), RNA-supplemented mice with induced tumors lived significantly longer than controls that did not receive RNA. It was suggested that the RNA was stimulating the animals' immunity against the tumors. This helped lead to a clinical human trial (*American Journal of Surgery*, 132:631, 1976) of "immune RNA," a preparation of RNA extracts of animal lymphoid tissues. Findings were inconclusive, but follow-up appears warranted.

By far the most interesting work in this area has been done with a *synthetic* polyribonucleotide, that is, a synthetic nucleic acid. Lacoue and co-workers (*Lancet*, July 26, 1980, p. 161) reported that Poly A/Poly U was useful in the treatment of women with breast cancers that had been operated upon. Some 300 patients were divided into two groups. The experimentals (155 women) received 30 milligrams of Poly A/Poly U intravenously each week for six weeks. The controls (145 women) received placebos (saline injections) on the same schedule. Follow-up over fifty months revealed a statistically significant increase in survival time among the experimentals—those who had been injected with Poly A/Poly U. No such increase was seen among the controls. No adverse side effects were noted. "Thus," these researchers concluded, "immunotherapy with Poly A/Poly U appears to be a simple, non-toxic, and efficient adjuvant treatment in operable breast cancer." The immune-stimulating effects of this complex had previously been noted in numerous animal studies (many of which are cited in the Lacoue paper). These are exciting findings but they require confirmation by others. Meanwhile, consumers are reminded that *no positive effects whatsoever have been noted in humans taking the RNA/DNA supplements available in vitamin stores.*

Claims are being made that RNA supplements can enhance memory and learning processes in various animals, including man. Cameron and colleagues (*American Journal of Psychiatry*, 120:320, 1963) found that RNA *injections* were of some benefit in the treatment of senile and arteriosclerotic dementias. Later, however, these same researchers (see review by Enesco, *Canadian Psychiatric Association Journal*, 12:29, 1967) found that RNA is *not* incorporated into brain tissue. The hypothesis thereafter was that some breakdown product of RNA is responsible for the observed therapeutic effects. Research has continued (see review by Lehmann and Ban in *Aging*, 2:149, 1975) but so far the results have not been promising. There is *no evidence whatever that oral RNA supplements have any beneficial effects on memory or learning in humans.*

There is some very preliminary evidence (*Mechanisms of Ageing and Development,* 17:283, 1981) that RNA has antioxidant properties. No conclusions can be drawn from this single report.

Users of oral RNA/DNA supplements may, particularly if they use these substances in high doses for prolonged periods, develop potentially dangerous hyperuricemia (excessive uric acid in the blood) and/or promote or aggravate gout.

My recommendation is to completely avoid RNA/DNA supplements.

Nucleic-Acid Derivatives of Current Experimental Interest

ADENOSINE

A number of claims have been made for adenosine and adenosine derivatives based largely upon uncontrolled, anecdotal European studies. One researcher has reported reductions in serum cholesterol and triglycerides following several weeks of treatment with a combination of oral and injected adenosine. Adenosine-treated patients with angina were said to obtain pain relief and, in about half the cases, objective EKG improvement. Some earlier studies reported adenosine to be of benefit in congestive heart failure (*Hippokrates,* 39:480, 1965) and in reducing the death rate from recurrent heart attack. Stone has recently reviewed the role of various adenosines in the nervous system (*Neuroscience,* 6:523, 1981). Disturbances in adenosine function may contribute to some nervous disorders, principally muscular dystrophy, but there is no convincing evidence that adenosine supplements, in any form, can be of benefit in these diseases. Supplementation is not recommended.

INOSINE AND DERIVATIVES

Some French doctors have reported that injected inosine is beneficial in the treatment of cardiac insufficiency, angina and senility. Wickham and colleagues (*British Medical Journal*, 2:173, 1978) reported on "the successful use of inosine in perfusing the kidney during conservative renal surgery in five patients." Another paper (*Cancer Treatment Reports*, 62:1963, 1978) reports on several studies demonstrating an antiviral activity of an inosine derivative—particularly against "slow virus" infections. (This derivative is isoprinosine.) Far more research will have to be done before any firm therapeutic claims for inosine can be justified. Supplementation is not recommended.

OROTATE

O'Sullivan (*Australian and New Zealand Journal of Medicine*, 3:417, 1973) has reviewed reports in which oral orotate was given with reported benefit in the treatment of various disorders, including heart attack, pernicious anemia and jaundice in the newborn. Russian studies (*Kardiologiia*, 6:54, 1966; *American Heart Journal*, 86:117, 1973) have reported orotate benefits in post-heart-attack treatment. More recently, Bailey (in Shibata and Bailey, eds., *Recent Developments in Cardiac Muscle Pharmacology*, Igaku-Shoin, Tokyo, 1982) has shown that orotic acid increases the strength of contractions of damaged cardiac muscle of dystrophic hamsters and concludes that orotic acid may have some future use in the management of congestive heart failure in humans, particularly since it is relatively nontoxic compared to the currently used drugs, such as digitalis. None of these studies is conclusive. At present, supplementation with orotate is *not* recommended.

eight

LIPIDS AND DERIVATIVES

Lipids represent a group of biological components that, in contrast to proteins and carbohydrates, are defined according to their solubility rather than their chemical structure. Of all the biological substances, the lipids are those that are least soluble in water. Substances classified as lipids include: triglycerides (fats), phospholipids, cholesterol, fatty acids and prostaglandins. The fatty acid linoleic acid is considered essential in that we cannot synthesize this substance and therefore have an absolute requirement for it in our diets.

High cholesterol levels are associated with an increased incidence of coronary heart disease and heart attacks. Diets of Western societies have had a tendency to be high in fats, cholesterol and fatty acids, especially of the saturated types (stearic and palmitic). We now know that increased intake of fatty acids of the mono-unsaturated types (palmitoleic, oleic) and especially of the *polyunsaturated* types (linoleic, linolenic) can *lower* serum cholesterol levels and so protect against coronary heart disease. Further, the long-chain fatty acids, found in cold-water oily fish, such as eicosapentaenoic acid (EPA) and docosahexaenoic acid (DHA), appear to inhibit the formation of the prostaglandin thromboxane in blood platelets. The decreased aggregation (clumping together) of platelets resulting from this is expected also to be beneficial in the prevention of coronary heart disease.

Choline/Lecithin

I. Overview

Lecithin has been a popular dietary supplement for many years. Pure lecithin is a phospholipid that is composed of saturated, unsaturated and/or polyunsaturated fatty acids. It also contains glycerin, phosphorus and a nitrogen-containing substance called choline. Lecithin is found in many foods and is of vital importance in cell-membrane structure; it acts as a bridge, allowing passage of substances into cells. This bridging capacity is related to lecithin's ability to associate with both water and lipids (substances not soluble in water).

Lecithin is a food additive found in ice cream, margarine and mayonnaise among others. It is the bridge that joins water to the fats in these products and thus helps maintain their consistency. It is one of the few truly nutritious agents used as a food additive. It is also a protector against oxidant damage.

There are many forms of lecithin—each form is characterized by the nature of the fatty acid it contains. The majority of lecithin products sold commercially do not contain pure lecithin; they contain such substances as inositol, which is not, contrary to popular belief, part of the structure of pure lecithin (see discussion of inositol).

Lecithin in food is the major source of the nutrient choline. Choline is extremely important for human health. In addition to contributing to the structure of lecithin, choline is involved in the synthesis of many important substances in the body; it is the precursor of acetylcholine, a molecule fundamental to the proper functioning of the nervous system. Acetylcholine is one of the neurotransmitters that determine human behavior. Alzheimer's disease, a presenile dementia characterized by deterioration of memory, judgment and orientation, appears to be due in part to a relative deficiency of acetylcholine in the brain. Attempts to treat Alzheimer's with supplemental choline have met with mixed to disappointing results to date; the work, however, is still in a very early stage and with modifications may yet prove to be of some benefit.

II. Claims

POSITIVE:
1) Protects against cardiovascular disease; 2) protects against memory loss and diseases of the nervous system.

III. Evidence

RELATED TO POSITIVE CLAIMS:

1) Protects against cardiovascular disease—This is a relatively old claim, though one that has persisted. It is based on findings that choline is involved in lipid metabolism in animals. There is no strong evidence, however, that *supplementary* choline affects lipid metabolism in humans. And the evidence that lecithin can favorably modify blood lipid levels is inconsistent. For a review of the pertinent literature, which shows that these substances can *raise*, as well as lower, blood lipids under varying circumstances, see Zeisel (*Annual Review of Nutrition*, 1:95, 1981). The evidence is somewhat more consistent, on the other hand, that *intravenous* choline can lower blood pressure in humans and a variety of other animals (see, for example, *Journal of Neurosurgery*, 32:468, 1970). Less significant results have been noted in this regard with oral choline. Further research will have to be done before the therapeutic role, if any, of choline and lecithin in cardiovascular disease can be clarified.

2) Protects against memory loss and diseases of the nervous system—Choline/lecithin have now been used in the experimental treatment of a number of neurological disorders. The results with respect to Alzheimer's disease have been regarded as "disappointing" by some researchers (*Lancet*, Nov. 27, 1982, p. 200) who had hoped that choline/lecithin might be to this disorder what L-dopa, for example, had been to Parkinson's. Still, even here the news has not been all bad.

Sufferers of Alzheimer's have exhibited a reduced ability to synthesize the chemical acetylcholine, which is required for the proper transmission of nerve impulses, especially, it appears, in those areas of the cerebral cortex associated with memory. This being the case, researchers hoped that supplemental choline/lecithin might boost acetylcholine activity in victims of Alzheimer's disease and thus improve their memories. And, in fact, there *is* evidence that such supplementation improves short-term memory in *some* of these patients (*Annals of Neurology*, 6:219, 1979). But there is no evidence that it can significantly arrest or reverse the disease. Recently, investigators at the Texas Research Institute of Mental Science in Houston found that lecithin seemed to improve the condition of patients with advanced Alzheimer's while worsening the condition of those with early manifestations of the disease (see report in *American Health*, Oct. 1983, p. 12). It is clear that claims going the rounds in the health-food circuit that lecithin and/or choline can prevent or even cure this frightening disease are unfounded. Further research with these substances may, however, help contribute to the solution to this disorder.

A study by Bartus and co-workers (*Science*, 209:301, 1980) found evidence of choline-induced memory enhancement in mice. Choline-enriched diet improved memory in the animals, while choline-deficient diets seemed to contribute to memory loss. Healthy humans given drugs that suppress acetylcholine activity have been shown to develop impaired short-term memory, while others given supplemental choline exhibit increased short-term memory skills (see Zeisel review cited above).

Cohen and colleagues (*American Journal of Psychiatry*, 137:242, 1980) found that lecithin administered in conjunction with lithium reduced manic episodes, which worsened again in 75 percent of the patients tested when lecithin, but not lithium, was withdrawn. Gelenberg and collaborators (*American Journal of Psychiatry*, 136:772, 1979) are among those who have reported that lecithin can, in some instances, significantly suppress the symptoms of tardive dyskinesia, an increasingly prevalent and serious neurological disorder that is one of the possible side effects of neuroleptic drugs used in the treatment of various psychological disorders: the disorder is characterized by twitching, jerking movements of the facial muscles and sometimes of the muscles in the trunk and extremities. So far, lecithin is the most effective treatment for this disorder. (It should be understood that the effect of lecithin in these studies is to supply choline.)

It appears that choline/lecithin play significant roles in a variety of neurological processes, especially memory. Research is continuing.

IV. Recommendations

A) SUGGESTED INTAKE: Optimal intake is unknown. Most Americans get between 400 and 900 milligrams of choline daily in their diet. This corresponds to about 4 to 9 grams of lecithin. Signs of dietary deficiency states have not been described, suggesting that average dietary intake may be adequate. Further research is required to determine how much choline we really need for optimal health.

B) SOURCE/FORM: Lecithin, and hence choline, is found in all animal and plant products. The foods richest in lecithin include egg yolks, soybeans, liver, cauliflower and cabbage. It is recommended that these foods be included in your diet. Those with high cholesterol levels who are restricting their intake of egg yolks (which, in fact, they should be doing) can increase their lecithin intake by eating more cauliflower and cabbage. I don't recommend nondietary choline/lecithin supplements; neither, however, do I see any reason to discourage those who are taking lecithin supplements (the best form of dietary choline) from doing so if they feel it is helping them. Some benefits may be possible even though they have not yet been clearly proved. But do not take more than 1,000 milligrams (1 gram) of supplemental choline daily or more than 10 grams of lecithin daily. Very high doses of oral choline have produced nausea, vomiting and dizziness in some people (taking up to 20 grams daily for several weeks); others on high doses have reported a fishy odor due to bacterial degradation of the choline in the intestine. Treatment of Alzheimer's disease with lecithin/choline should be done only under a physician's supervision.

Individuals who are taking megadoses of vitamin B_3 (nicotinic acid/niacin) for the treatment of high serum lipids (cholesterol and triglycerides) should have a lecithin-rich diet or take a choline supplement of 1,000 milligrams daily (or 10 grams of lecithin daily). Rats fed a choline-poor diet developed problems related to methyl-donation reactions, which are very important biochemical events in cellular growth. Nicotinic acid can trap methyl groups and make them inaccessible biochemically. The dose used in these experiments corresponds to a human dose of 9 grams of nicotinic acid daily—a dose some patients do use (*Journal of Nutrition*, 113:315, 1983). But, except for these individuals, there is no specific indication, based on current knowledge, for choline/lecithin supplementation.

EPA/MaxEPA (Fish Oils/Marine Lipids)

I. Overview

Eicosapentaenoic acid (EPA) is a long-chain fatty acid that affects the synthesis of prostaglandins, a complex family of hormonelike substances that have far-reaching regulatory effects in the body. It has been touted as a potent protective agent against various forms of cardiovascular disease. The claims made for EPA are supported by scientific evidence. EPA, in fact, is causing quite a stir in the medical community.

Much of the excitement is due to the epidemiological studies of Eskimos and of Japanese, who consume large quantities of fish and other marine life rich in EPA. Both groups studied are at significantly lower risk than most other populations of suffering from various heart and circulatory disorders, which are among the major killers of modern times. Clinical studies have also shown EPA-related protective effects, though the long-term studies that are required to confirm these are still under way. Such are the hopes inspired by research to date that normally circumspect medical magazines and journals have quipped "A salmon a day may keep a coronary away" (*Medical World News*, Jan. 18, 1982) and run such headlines as "It's Not Fishy: Fruit of the Sea May Foil Cardiovascular Disease" (*Journal of American Medical Association*, Feb. 12, 1982). Whether all of this exuberance is entirely justified remains to be conclusively demonstrated. Meanwhile, there are some dangers in megadosing on fish oil, as discussed below.

II. Claims

POSITIVE:
1) Protects against cardiovascular disease; 2) protects against arthritis.

NEGATIVE:
1) Toxic; 2) large doses may diminish immunity and predispose to some cancers.

III. Evidence

RELATED TO POSITIVE CLAIMS:

1) Protects against cardiovascular disease—It is a striking fact that, despite a diet high in protein, fat and cholesterol and very low in carbohydrate, fiber and vitamin C, many Eskimos have a remarkably low incidence of blood clots, narrowing of the arteries, heart attacks and other manifestations of cardiovascular disease (*Acta Medica Scandinavica*, 200:69, 1976; and review, *Lancet*, May 21, 1983, p. 1139). Greenland Eskimos, whose diet consists primarily of fish, seal and whale meat, have low blood levels of triglycerides and total cholesterol, high levels of high-density lipoprotein (HDL) cholesterol, which is known to have a cardiovascular protective effect, and decreased platelet aggregation, which makes them resistant to clotting disorders (*Lancet*, 2:117, 1978). In coastal villages of Japan where fish is the main dietary staple, similar epidemiological findings have been noted (*Lancet*, 2:1132, 1980; *Lancet*, 2:197, 1981).

The primary protective component of this diet has been identified as EPA, which is believed to exert its favorable effects through prostaglandin activity (*Lancet*, June 5, 1982, p. 1269). Among other things, EPA inhibits prostaglandin effects that promote blood-clotting mechanisms.

There have been numerous clinical studies (see review in *Medical Letter*, 24:99, 1982) designed to investigate the possible cardioprotective effects of fish diets, fish oils and EPA supplements. Most of these human studies have shown some favorable effects. Goodnight and co-workers, for example, reported (*Blood*, 58:880, 1981) that 11 healthy volunteers who derived most of their fats and cholesterol from a diet of salmon exhibited signs suggestive of clot resistance and had decreased cholesterol concentrations; these improvements were evident four weeks after starting the salmon diet. Similar findings were noted by Sanders and group (*Clinical Science*, 61:317, 1981) using a cod-liver-oil preparation that provided 1.8 grams per day of EPA and 2.2 grams per day of a related fatty acid and by Hay and co-workers (*Lancet*, 1:1269, 1982) using a fish oil that supplied 3.5 grams per day of EPA.

Saynor and Verel (*Lancet*, June 11, 1983, p. 1335) report that they have studied the effects in humans of MaxEPA (trade name for a fish-oil preparation, sold in health-food stores under various labels, containing EPA and a related fatty acid called docosahexaenoic acid—DHA) since 1980 and have followed some 150 subjects who have taken it for up to three years. Many of these subjects had previously suffered heart attacks or were currently experiencing angina or other manifestations of cardio-vascular disease. Some of the favorable results noted declined over time, but others persisted even after two years.

As yet, though, there have been no long-term double-blind, placebo-controlled studies of the effects of EPA in humans. Results to date are promising enough to indicate that these more elaborate studies should be carried out to provide more conclusive information. Some are under way now.

2) Protects against arthritis—There is no evidence to support this claim, although Ziff (*Arthritis and Rheumatism*, 26:457, 1983) has suggested that a diet rich in EPA might inhibit the production of certain prostaglandins implicated in inflammatory processes seen in some forms of arthritis. Investigation is warranted.

RELATED TO NEGATIVE CLAIMS:

1) Toxic—Fish oils contain almost no vitamin C or E; thus they peroxidize (become rancid) easily and quickly. Moreover, the fish oils that contain EPA also contain cetoleic acid, which has been shown to be toxic in the cardiac (heart) muscle of some animals (*Progress in the Chemistry of Fats and the Other Lipids*, 15:29, 1977). Mackerel-oil supplements resulted in some liver damage in pigs (*American Journal of Clinical Nutrition*, 31:2159, 1978). Goodnight (cited above) noted that some of the individuals studied who were on diets high in fish oils/EPA ex-

hibited thrombocytopenia, a persistent decrease in blood platelets. This decrease might be desirable in persons with a tendency to form inappropriate blood clots but not so desirable in healthy people. Thrombocytopenia is seen in hemorrhage. Saynor and Verel, however, have noted (cited above) that the level of cetoleic acid in the MaxEPA preparations widely available is less than 2 percent. Many of these preparations come mixed with vitamin E, which helps protect against rancidity. Nonetheless, some individuals might encounter problems with even small concentrations of cetoleic acid, particularly if megadoses of EPA are taken on a regular basis. Bleeding problems might also arise under these circumstances.

2) Large doses may diminish immunity and predispose to some cancers—A possible relationship between highly unsaturated fats and diminished immune function has been suggested (*Medical Letter*, cited above), and development of malignancy, associated with reduced immunity and/or other factors, is under investigation (see *Diet, Nutrition and Cancer*, National Research Council, National Academy Press, Washington, D.C., 1982). There is also some evidence contradicting the above; there is, in any event, no evidence that moderate dietary intake diminishes immunity or predisposes to cancer.

IV. Recommendations

I do not recommend that you take EPA/MaxEPA or other fish-oil supplements. As noted above, fish oils are particularly prone to rancidity. In addition, these supplements invite overdosing, which may expose you to some of the potentially serious perils discussed above. The epidemiological evidence of EPA-related cardioprotective effects, however, is exciting. My recommendation is that you include in your diet, on a regular basis, such "oily" fish as salmon, cod and mackerel. Use supplements only if so directed by a physician.

Gamma-Linolenic Acid (And Oil of Evening Primrose)

I. Overview

The claims for oil of evening primrose (a particularly rich source of gamma-linolenic acid) seem almost boundless these days— despite a dearth of reliable research on the subject. In the tireless hyperbole of the "true believers," it is touted as another "miracle worker" that can cure everything from brittle nails to cancer. The Pilgrims are supposed to have been introduced to the herbal powers of this oil by the Indians; exported to England, the oil is said to have become known as the "King's Cure-All." The persistent claims have paid off—at least in the sense that science has started looking into the properties of this oil, but with decidedly mixed results.

The so-called "miracle ingredient" of oil of evening primrose is gamma-linolenic acid (GLA), which the body makes from essential fatty acids. Linolenic acid is the primary dietary source of the essential fatty acids, which have numerous functions in the body; among other things they are precursors of an important family of substances collectively known as the prostaglandins. There has been an explosion of research related to the prostaglandins in recent years, and it is now known that they have complex and profound effects throughout the body, such as regulation of platelet aggregation, blood vessel tone, salt and water balance, gastrointestinal function, neurotransmitter function and secretion of insulin. Linoleic acid is converted in the body to GLA, via enzymatic action, and thereafter can contribute to prostaglandin synthesis. Thus, the simplistic claim has been that the more GLA you get, the more prostaglandins you'll have and the healthier you will be in every respect. This claim overlooks the fact that we still have a great deal to learn about the prostaglandins; it also overlooks one very important thing we do know about them—that different varieties of prostaglandins have different and sometimes contrary effects. They can, for example, in their different forms, be both anti-inflammatory and pro-inflammatory; they can both increase and decrease platelet aggregation (blood-clotting factors). The ratios in which these "contrary" prostaglandins are actively expressed at any given time thus helps determine a complex set of biochemical events. Different prostaglandins can be both "good" and "bad" under varying circumstances.

In summary, more is not always better. Given our present level of knowledge, trying to "fine tune" our prostaglandin biochemistry with high daily doses of oil of evening primrose is a little like trying to modify a microchip with a hammer. It's not likely to be effective—except in carefully selected, medically monitored cases; and it might prove damaging.

II. Claims

POSITIVE:
1) Protects against cardiovascular disease; 2) heals eczema and improves other skin disorders; 3) fights cancer; 4) combats arthritis; 5) miscellaneous cure-all.

III. Evidence

RELATED TO POSITIVE CLAIMS:

1) Protects against cardiovascular disease—GLA is said to help prevent heart attacks by inhibiting blood clots and arterial spasms. It is true that various of the prostaglandins are active in the regulation of the cardiovascular system. Horrobin (*Medical Hypotheses*, 6:785, 1980) has argued that a decrease in one particular form of prostaglandin "will lead to a potentially catastrophic series of untoward consequences," including elevated cholesterol production, enhanced blood clotting and increased chance of heart attacks. He has also argued that GLA, in the form of oil of evening primrose, can help forestall these catastrophes. Unfortunately, sound published data are in short supply to either refute or support these claims. Research of a well-controlled nature is needed to test this interesting hypothesis.

2) Heals eczema and improves other skin disorders—Wright and Barton (*Lancet*, Nov. 20, 1982, p. 1120) reported significant

clinical improvement in a double-blind crossover study of 99 patients whose atopic eczema was treated with varying oral doses of evening-primrose oil. (Atopic eczema is an inflammatory disease of the skin of unknown etiology and is very resistant to treatment.) Chalmers and Shuster (*Lancet*, Jan. 29, 1983, p. 236), however, failed to note any therapeutic benefit in another double-blind study of 30 patients whose ichthyosis vulgaris (a hereditary skin disease characterized by dryness, roughness, scaliness) was treated with evening-primrose oil. A substantial number of these patients were also suffering from atopic eczema, and there was no significant improvement in that condition either.

Various modes of action by which GLA might modify prostaglandin activity in such a way that improvement might be seen in a number of skin disorders, including psoriasis, have been suggested (*Archives of Dermatology*, 119:541, 1983) but not demonstrated. As Hanifin recently observed (*Journal of the American Academy of Dermatology*, 8(5):729, 1983), "at present, the efficacy of evening-primrose oil in atopic dermatitis is unconfirmed and awaits the support of independent studies."

3) Fights cancer—There is no present evidence that GLA/oil of evening primrose has any beneficial effect in the treatment of cancer. However, some recent studies show that GLA selectively killed human esophageal carcinoma cells growing in tissue culture (*South African Medical Journal*, 62:505 and 681, 1982).

4) Combats arthritis—In a review of various dietary approaches to treating rheumatoid arthritis, Ziff (*Arthritis and Rheumatism*, 26:457, 1983) discusses some of the inflammatory and anti-inflammatory effects of the prostaglandins, as well as their impact on immunity and other factors that are thought to be involved in rheumatoid arthritis. Fatty acids are discussed and various types of experimentation are proposed. While there are insufficient data to justify current claims that GLA can have any impact on arthritis, research of this issue is warranted.

5) Miscellaneous cure-all—There are anecdotal or otherwise unsubstantiated claims that GLA is an aid in dieting, that it

improves the quality of the fingernails, is effective for hangovers and as a means of alleviating symptoms of premenstrual tension, that it is useful in the treatment of multiple sclerosis and for the management of hyperactive children. Claims that GLA may be useful in the treatment of schizophrenia similarly remain unsubstantiated.

IV. Recommendations

I do *not* recommend GLA/oil of evening primrose supplements. The claims made for these have not been substantiated. Instead, concentrate on cutting down on the saturated (largely animal) fats in your diet, and to the extent that you want to replace them with other fats, use polyunsaturated fats (most vegetable oils) for which lipid-lowering effects have been demonstrated. About 25 to 30 percent of your fatty-acid intake should be of the polyunsaturated variety.

Inositol
(Myo-inositol)

I. Overview

Like choline, myo-inositol, the biologically active form of inositol, is a constituent of phospholipids, those water-insoluble structures that are essential in cell membranes. Although clear-cut deficiency states have not been identified in humans, they have been described in some other animals. (See review by Kuskis and Mookerjea, *Nutrition Reviews*, 36:233, 1978.) Myo-inositol is recognized as important in the metabolism of fats, and it has long been claimed that it can lower blood concentrations of fats and cholesterol. The most significant findings with respect to myo-inositol, however, relate to diabetes, as discussed below.

II. Claims

POSITIVE:
1) Protects against cardiovascular disease; 2) protects against diabetes; 3) protects against hair loss.

III. Evidence

RELATED TO POSITIVE CLAIMS:

1) Protects against cardiovascular disease—Gavin and Mc-Henry were the first (*Journal of Biological Chemistry*, 139:485, 1941) to show that myo-inositol is a lipotropic agent (reducing the amount of fat in liver) in rats. Others (see Kuskis review cited above) have since confirmed and extended these findings. There is, however, no evidence that myo-inositol protects *humans* against cardiovascular disease. Research is needed to further explore the role of myo-inositol in human fat metabolism.

2) Protects against diabetes—While there is no evidence that myo-inositol can *prevent* diabetes, there is some worthwhile evidence suggesting that it may be useful in the treatment of diabetic peripheral neuropathy, one of the most crippling complications of this disease. It is now believed that decreased levels of myo-inositol in the nerves of diabetics suffering from this complication are associated with the damage to nerve fiber. The adverse effects of chronic high blood sugar on these fibers may be heightened by reduced myo-inositol concentrations in the nerves (*New England Journal of Medicine*, 308:152, 1983). Salway and co-workers (*Lancet*, 2:1282, 1978) found that myo-inositol given in doses of 500 milligrams twice a day for two weeks increased the amplitude of the evoked action potential of certain nerves, suggesting that a greater number of nerves were firing after stimulation. No such apparent improvement was noted when placebo was given. Clements and colleagues (*American Journal of Clinical Nutrition*, 33:1954, 1980) have reported improved sensory nerve function in 20 diabetic patients with neuropathy in whom dietary intake of myo-inositol was increased from 772 to 1,648 milligrams daily.

Further research is warranted to see whether myo-inositol does indeed play an important role in this disorder, its treatment and prevention. Research to date is promising but not yet conclusive.

3) Protects against hair loss—There is no evidence to support this claim.

IV. Recommendations

A) SUGGESTED INTAKE: Estimated intake in U.S. diet ranges from 300 to 1,000 milligrams of myo-inositol daily. Optimal intake remains unknown. There are indications that diabetic patients should plan their diets to ensure high intake of this substance (about 1,000 to 1,500 milligrams daily).

B) SOURCE/FORM: Myo-inositol is widely distributed in plant and animal products. Citrus fruits (except lemons) and cantaloupes are excellent sources of myo-inositol. For example, a quarter of a fresh cantaloupe of average size contains 355 milligrams; one orange contains 307 milligrams; one-half of a grapefruit has 200 milligrams; one-half cup of frozen concentrate of grapefruit contains 456 milligrams; one-half cup of frozen concentrate of orange has 245 milligrams; one slice of whole-wheat bread contains 288 milligrams. Beans, grains and nuts are also good sources.

I see no reason to take supplementary myo-inositol at this time. Toxicity of such supplements, however, is low. No side effects were observed in human subjects taking 3 grams of oral myo-inositol daily or 1 gram intravenously daily for short periods of time (Inositol, in *The Vitamins*, Vol. 3, 2nd ed., Academic Press, New York, 1971).

Consumers of inositol should be aware that *myo*-inositol is the only biologically active form of this compound.

Diabetics who take supplementary myo-inositol should do so under a physician's supervision.

nine

OTHER SUPPLEMENTS

Extensive anti-aging claims have been made—or are likely to be made—for a number of established and emerging food supplements that cannot be categorized as vitamins, minerals, amino acids, nucleic acids or lipids. The supplements analyzed in this chapter are:

L-Carnitine
Dietary Fiber
Garlic
Ginseng
Pangamic Acid
Superoxide Dismutase
Wheatgrass/Barley Grass

In addition, the following miscellaneous supplements are analyzed in a briefer, less formal fashion: acidophilus, aloe vera, bee pollen, bioflavonoids, brewer's yeast, capsicum, chondroitin sulfate, coenzyme Q, glandulars, PABA, royal jelly, spirulina, wheat germ, wheat-germ oil and octacosanol.

Pharmaceuticals and various other chemicals for which anti-aging claims have been made are analyzed in Chapter Ten.

L-Carnitine

I. Overview

Carnitine is a relative newcomer to the supplement market-place, but it is beginning to cause a bit of excitement. Chemically, carnitine is a quaternary amine (the same chemical family that includes choline) and exists as two stereoisomers (structures that are mirror images of each other) called L-carnitine (the active form found in our tissues) and D-carnitine (biologically inactive form). An equal mixture of the two forms is called DL-carnitine. L-carnitine is synthesized in the human body, chiefly in the liver and kidneys, from essential amino acids, lysine and methionine. Three vitamins, niacin, B_6 and C, as well as iron, are involved in this synthesis.

It is now established that L-carnitine is essential for the maintenance of good health in humans. (See excellent review of the carnitine literature by Borum, *Annual Review of Nutrition*, 3:233, 1983.) L-carnitine is absolutely necessary for the transport of long-chain fatty acids into the mitochondria, the metabolic furnaces of the cells. Fatty acids are the major sources for production of energy in the heart and skeletal muscles, structures that are particularly vulnerable to L-carnitine deficiency. A number of L-carnitine-deficiency states have now been identified, several of which are genetic in origin. Symptoms of such deficiencies include muscle weakness, severe confusion and angina ("heart pain").

There are a few groups at particular risk of L-carnitine deficiency. These include chronic-kidney-failure patients on hemodialysis and patients with liver failure. Even some healthy subgroups have additional needs for dietary L-carnitine. These include strict vegetarians, newborns, pregnant women and women who are nursing infants.

It has only recently been recognized that dietary L-carnitine is essential for optimal health. The future looks bright for this substance so long as medical science continues to investigate the possible roles it plays in the protection against age-associated disease.

II. Claims

POSITIVE:
1) Protects against cardiovascular disease; 2) protects against muscle disease (and helps build muscle and stamina); 3) protects against liver disease; 4) protects against diabetes; 5) protects against kidney disease; 6) aids in dieting.

NEGATIVE:
1) Causes muscle disease.

III. Evidence

RELATED TO POSITIVE CLAIMS:

1) Protects against cardiovascular disease—Clinical trials have demonstrated positive effects of L-carnitine supplementation in patients suffering from various forms of cardiovascular disease. Kosolcharoen and colleagues (*Current Therapeutic Research*, 30:753, 1981), for example, demonstrated significantly improved tolerance to exercise in patients suffering from coronary-artery disease who were given intravenous L-carnitine. Thomsen and co-workers (*American Journal of Cardiology*, 43:300, 1979) have also demonstrated increased tolerance to exercise among L-carnitine-treated patients with coronary-artery disease. In another study (*International Journal of Tissue Reactions*, 11:175, 1980), two matched groups of patients suffering from angina pectoris (the severe chest pain that often accompanies insufficient flow of blood and oxygen to the heart muscle) were given two different forms of carnitine. Notable improvement was observed in both groups during the first thirty days in which oral carnitine was provided. Between thirty and sixty days, however, *further* improvement was observed in the group receiving L-carnitine (50 milligrams per kilogram of body weight daily) but *not* in the group receiving DL-carnitine (100 milligrams per kilogram of body weight daily). (See Overview and Recommendations for more on the different forms of carnitine.)

It was reported some time ago that supplemental carnitine

can significantly reduce total blood lipids (fats and fatlike substances), a finding confirmed in recent years by Japanese researchers who reported (*Lancet*, 1:805, 1978) that giving 900 milligrams per day of oral L-carnitine could notably reduce levels of blood triglycerides, which are among the lipids implicated in cardiovascular disease. Oral L-carnitine, in this trial, was as effective as intravenous L-carnitine. The lowering effect continued so long as L-carnitine was supplied; triglyceride levels rose again when carnitine was withdrawn. No effect was noted on cholesterol. However, in another study (*Johns Hopkins Medical Journal*, 150:51, 1982), 1 gram of oral L-carnitine administered daily over a period of ten to fifteen weeks produced a substantial increase in high-density lipoprotein (HDL) cholesterol in two normal men. HDL is the "good" cholesterol, the part that is *protective* against coronary-artery disease.

Research to date thus suggests a potentially important role for L-carnitine in the treatment and possibly the prevention of some forms of cardiovascular disease. There is no evidence at present, however, to suggest that persons with *normal* carnitine levels and normal fatty-acid metabolism will benefit from non-dietary carnitine supplementation. Further research is warranted.

2) Protects against muscle disease (and helps build muscle and stamina)—Patients with some forms of muscle-weakening diseases, most of which are hereditary, have been shown to have carnitine deficiencies that in some instances respond to carnitine supplementation. (See review of Rebouche and Engel, *Mayo Clinic Proceedings*, 58:533, 1983.) Claims that carnitine can help build muscle and increase physical endurance have led to the use of this substance by some athletes and body-builders. It is possible that normal individuals may derive some energy-enhancing benefits from carnitine supplements, but there is no proof that this is the case.

3) Protects against liver disease—There is little evidence that carnitine is directly protective against liver disease. Carnitine deficiencies, however, may disturb the normal processes of liver metabolism of lipoproteins, contributing to potentially dangerous elevations in blood levels of triglycerides and cholesterol. (See discussion of cardiovascular disease above.)

4) Protects against diabetes—Though abnormalities of carnitine metabolism have been reported in diabetics, there is no proof that supplemental carnitine will prevent diabetes.

5) Protects against kidney disease—This claim apparently arises from reports (such as *Lancet,* 1:882, 1979) that the now often-noted carnitine deficiency of kidney patients undergoing hemodialysis could be prevented via oral carnitine supplementation. There is no evidence, however, that such supplements will benefit *normal* individuals who seek to prevent the development of kidney disorders.

6) Aids in dieting—McCarty (*Medical Hypotheses,* 8:269, 1982) has suggested that carnitine might be a useful supplement for those who are on low-calorie diets. He hypothesizes that carnitine, by enhancing the efficiency of fatty-acid oxidation (increasing the burn rate of calories stored as fat), may make low-calorie diets easier to tolerate by reducing feelings of hunger and weakness that result from less efficient oxidation of fats. This is an intriguing hypothesis worthy of some investigation.

RELATED TO NEGATIVE CLAIMS:

1) Causes muscle disease—Symptoms of myasthenia (progressive weakness of certain muscle groups without evidence of atrophy or wasting) have been reported (*Lancet,* 1:1041, 1979; *Journal of the Neurological Sciences,* 46:365, 1980) in kidney patients being maintained for prolonged periods of time on hemodialysis and supplemental DL-carnitine. Symptoms disappeared upon withdrawal of the DL-carnitine. When, at a later date, these same patients were given the L-form of carnitine (L-carnitine), the myasthenia symptoms did *not* return (*Lancet,* 1:1209, 1979). These findings suggest that supplements should be in the form of L-carnitine and *not* in the form of the presently marketed DL-carnitine.

IV. Recommendations

A) SUGGESTED INTAKE: The dietary intake of L-carnitine for optimal health is unknown. In fact, the amount of L-carnitine in the average Western diet remains undefined. An unpublished analysis (see the review of Borum, cited above) of hospitalized patients in the United States showed dietary intake of between 2 (two) and 300 milligrams daily while on hospital diet. No recommendation can be made until more—and better—information is at hand.

B) SOURCE/FORM: Dietary sources richest in L-carnitine are red meats (lamb and beef in particular). Dairy products contain some L-carnitine. Vegetables, fruits and certain cereals contain little or no L-carnitine. (Avocados have some; so does the fermented soybean product tempeh.)

C) TAKE WITH: Supplements not recommended at this time.

D) CAUTIONARY NOTE: Be aware that the only supplemental form of carnitine on the market at this writing is the DL-form. This form has been shown to cause a myasthenia-type syndrome (see Evidence: Related to Negative Claims above) in some patients. The L-carnitine form, on the other hand, has *not* produced negative side effects, even in some individuals taking 1.6 grams daily for more than one year (*Current Therapeutic Research*, 31:1042, 1982).

Dietary Fiber

I. Overview

Despite the fact that dietary fiber contains no nutrients, it is rapidly coming to be recognized as a very important food constituent. It has, in effect, recently become a major food supplement—and with good reason. The literature now abounds with evidence suggesting substantial and often surprising health benefits of fiber. Previously, fiber was dismissed as "unassimilable carbohydrates" or as "mere roughage." Though many have heard that fiber may protect against some forms of cancer, far fewer are aware of other, perhaps better, evidence suggesting that fiber may lower blood pressure, reduce the risk of coronary heart disease and help control diabetes and obesity.

Dietary fiber, for the most part, is made up of indigestible portions of plant cells called polysaccharides. These polysaccharides, of which there is a variety, help form the structure of plant-cell walls; they are the very substance of plant architecture. Cereals, vegetables and fruits are important sources of dietary fiber. Up until the early 1970s, foods were increasingly being processed to rid them of fiber; even today dietary intake of fiber is much lower in the U.S. than it was a hundred years ago.

What I call "fiber-consciousness" began growing soon after Burkitt published a significant paper (*Lancet*, 2:1229, 1969) in which he suggested that the low incidence of cancer of the colon and rectum among those living in tropical parts of Africa might well be due to their high intake of dietary fiber. Burkitt's data commanded attention, particularly in the U.S. and Europe, where the incidence of intestinal cancer was high and rising and the intake of dietary fiber was low and getting lower. The rest, as they say, is history, though history still in the making. A great deal still remains to be learned about dietary fiber and its effects in the body. Some of its alleged benefits, though certainly suggested by the available data, remain unproved in the strictest sense.

Although dietary fiber is not a nutrient in the conventional sense, there is increasing evidence that a high-dietary-fiber intake is essential for the maintenance of optimal health. Dietary fiber may be most important in controlling the rate of entrance (absorption) of glucose into the bloodstream. A fast rate of glucose absorption conceivably plays a significant role in some of the disease processes associated with aging, such as cardiovascular disease and cancer.

II. Claims

POSITIVE:
1) Protects against cancer and other diseases of the colon and rectum; 2) effective in the treatment of diabetes; 3) capable of lowering cholesterol and blood pressure; 4) effective in weight-reduction diets.

NEGATIVE:
1) Causes gas and diarrhea; 2) can obstruct the small intestine; 3) causes mineral deficiencies.

III. Evidence

RELATED TO POSITIVE CLAIMS:

1) Protects against cancer and other diseases of the colon and rectum—Soon after Burkitt's startling report appeared in 1969 (cited in Overview above), Painter (*British Medical Journal*, 2:156, 1971) further upset orthodox thinking about fiber when he reported that symptoms of diverticular disease of the colon (small herniations through the wall of the intestine) could be treated with considerable success by a diet high in fiber. This flew in the face of the then prevailing—but usually unsatisfactory—treatment with bland *low-fiber* diet. The preferred treatment for the symptoms of diverticular disease, the incidence of which increases with age, is now 15 to 30 grams daily of supplemental fiber, usually in the form of coarse wheat bran (which also takes care of any constipation). It is *probable* that increasing intake of dietary fiber will help protect against the development of this disorder.

Meanwhile, claims that dietary fiber protects against cancers of the colon and rectum, though supported by some of the epidemiological data, remain unproved. Eastwood and Passmore, in an excellent review (*Lancet*, July 23, 1983, p. 202) of the dietary-fiber literature, point out that many foods contain traces of cancer-causing chemicals that are more likely to do damage the longer they are retained in the intestines. "A possible explanation," they write, "of the lower incidence of carcinoma of the colon and rectum in Africa than in Europe and North America is that high-fibre diets by reducing transit time and diluting faecal constituents reduce exposure to unidentified carcinogens." In short, increased fiber intake may more quickly rid our "systems" of some cancer-causing substances known to be present in our diets. (See *Science*, 221:1256, 1983.)

2) Effective in the treatment of diabetes—In 1976, Kiehm and co-workers (*American Journal of Clinical Nutrition*, 29:895, 1976) launched the high-carbohydrate, high-fiber diet in the management of insulin-treated diabetic patients. They reported substantial reductions (25 to 50 percent) in the need for insulin among diabetes mellitus patients placed on this diet. Others

(*British Medical Journal*, 2:523, 1979; *Diabetes Care*, 5:529, 1982) confirmed these findings. Anderson and Ward (*American Journal of Clinical Nutrition*, 32:2312, 1979) have also reported that a high-fiber diet (65 grams of plant fiber daily) reduces insulin requirements. The only adverse side effect noted was "tolerable" increased gas in the intestines.

Anderson and group acknowledge that the mechanisms by which their diet benefits diabetics remain poorly understood but note that dietary fiber slows the digestion and absorption of carbohydrates and may thus decrease the rise in blood levels of sugar following meals. More recent studies continue to support an essential role for a high intake of dietary fiber in the management of diabetic patients (*Acta Medica Scandinavica*, Supplement 671:87, 91, 1983). The available data in support of a role for dietary fiber in the treatment of diabetes are strong enough that the National Diabetes Associations of the U.S., Canada, Great Britain and Australia have all endorsed high-fiber diet (*Diabetes Care*, 5:59, 1982).

3) Capable of lowering cholesterol and blood pressure—Anderson and co-workers (cited above) found that *water-soluble* (but not insoluble) fibers, of the sort derived from oat products and dried beans, could lower those constituents of cholesterol that have been implicated in atherosclerosis (narrowing of arteries due to fatty deposits). Kirby, Anderson et al. (*American Journal of Clinical Nutrition*, 34:824, 1981) observed a 13 percent reduction in serum cholesterol in patients with abnormally high cholesterol levels. This reduction occurred over a thirteen-day period in which 100 grams of fiber were added to diet daily, either in the form of oat bran (one bowl of cereal and five oat muffins) or dried beans (four daily servings of navy or pinto beans). Considerably larger reductions were noted in subsequent work by Anderson and others over longer periods of time. (High-density lipoprotein—HDL—cholesterol, which is considered *protective* against atherosclerosis, *increased* under the apparent influence of dietary fiber, while the disease-contributing low-density cholesterol levels *decreased*.) Further research is definitely warranted to determine the long-term role of high dietary fiber in lowering cholesterol levels.

There is less evidence (*Annals of Internal Medicine*, 98:842, 1983) that fiber can reduce blood pressure, but this claim too deserves further research.

4) Effective in weight-reduction diets—Anderson and Sieling (*Obesity and Bariatric Medicine*, 9:109, 1980) reported that in a crossover study of obese diabetic patients an 800-calorie high-fiber diet produced a significantly greater sense of fullness and less hunger than did an 800-calorie low-fiber diet. Eastwood and Passmore (cited above) note that the higher bulk of high-fiber foods (which also require more chewing) might be expected to have some impact on obesity. As of now, however, this claim remains unproved. Long-term studies will be required to determine whether fiber can make weight loss less temporary and less a chore than it is for most dieters today.

RELATED TO NEGATIVE CLAIMS:

1) Causes gas and diarrhea—Abdominal distress is common among those who make large, abrupt additions of fiber to their diets. Even then most individuals adjust to the increased fiber over a period of a few weeks. The best approach is to increase fiber intake *gradually*.

2) Can obstruct the small intestine—This occurs, but only very rarely. Likelihood of obstruction is increased if there is some preexisting inflammation, as in the case of Crohn's disease. Individuals with diseases of the bowels should consult their doctors to determine the best amount of fiber in their diets.

3) Causes mineral deficiencies—Extremely high fiber intake has been associated with various mineral deficiencies. Fiber binds to minerals and may impair their absorption to some extent and increase their excretion via the feces. Eastwood and Passmore (cited above) write: "It can be stated with confidence that people who increase their fiber intake up to 50 grams a day, double the amount usually present in British [and U.S.] diets, run no risk of any serious adverse effects on their health." Actually, though, there are very few studies on the specific effects of high-dietary-fiber intake on mineral absorption. Such studies are warranted in view of the fact that marginal mineral deficiencies are possible with increased fiber intake. (See discussion of minerals elsewhere in this book, specifically calcium, iron and zinc.) It seems likely, in any event, that if there is a problem the solution is not to reduce fiber intake but to increase mineral intake.

IV. Recommendations

A) SUGGESTED INTAKE: The dietary intake for optimal longevity and health is not presently known. The evidence suggests that this figure is somewhere between 40 to 60 grams daily. Vegetarians may already be getting 40 grams or more daily. Some individuals, who favor low-fiber processed foods, may be getting only 10 grams of fiber per day. It is generally believed that fiber intake in the U.S. and Europe is too low.

B) SOURCE/FORM: Eastwood and Passmore (cited above) observe that the average 25 grams per day of fiber consumed by individuals in the U.S., Britain and much of Europe are derived from bread and cereal products (10 grams), potatoes (7 grams), other vegetables (6 grams) and fruit (2 grams). This is the *average* fiber intake; many Americans consume far less. There are a number of bran cereals, high in fiber, on the market today. Check labels for fiber content. Dried beans are a good source of fiber. Others are rice, especially brown rice, and whole-grain breads and bran muffins. One slice of whole-wheat bread contains 5 grams of bran. Bran is the best source of dietary fiber. About 50 percent of bran is fiber.

C) TAKE WITH: Adequate minerals, the absorption of which may be impaired in some cases when dietary-fiber intake is quite high; best to take these minerals in a well-balanced vitamin/mineral "insurance" formula. (See Part Three for more specific recommendations.)

D) CAUTIONARY NOTE: Diabetic patients requiring insulin would like nothing more than to stop sticking themselves with needles every day. Sadly, I have treated patients in the intensive-care unit who have decided to stop their insulin because a product available in the supplement marketplace was touted as a "cure" for diabetes. Dietary fiber *is* important in the management of diabetes mellitus, but it is not a cure-all. Patients who increase their intake of dietary fiber should not assume that they can forget about insulin injections but, rather, should collaborate very closely with their physicians regarding the precise amount of insulin required in conjunction with fiber diet.

Garlic
(With a Note on
Onions)

I. Overview

Garlic has long been a sturdy staple of health-food stores. It seems to be everyone's favorite "folk remedy" for just about everything that ails mankind. *Allium sativum*—garlic—is a common plant used to spice foods throughout the world. Probably the most substantial claim that has been made for garlic is that it can reduce cholesterol levels and help protect against narrowing of the arteries. To the surprise of many researchers, garlic is exhibiting some potentially important effects in current studies.

II. Claims

POSITIVE:
1) Protects against atherosclerosis and coronary-artery disease; 2) has antibiotic effects; 3) protects against cancer; 4) increases energy.

NEGATIVE:
1) Toxic; 2) offensive.

III. Evidence

RELATED TO POSITIVE CLAIMS:

1) Protects against atherosclerosis and coronary-artery disease —Lau and colleagues (*Nutrition Research*, 3:119, 1983) have recently reviewed the world literature related to research on garlic's effect on factors known to contribute to narrowing of the arteries (atherosclerosis). Their conclusions: "The positive reports appear to be overwhelming. The reviewers were surprised by the scarcity of negative reports." They review a variety of animal studies, some well controlled, in which garlic clearly exhibited a statistically significant lowering effect on the components of cholesterol that are associated with increased risk of

heart disease. In most of the studies the cholesterol-lowering effects of garlic were "dose-related," meaning that the higher the daily dose of garlic, the greater the reduction in cholesterol (see, for example, *Atherosclerosis*, 29:125, 1978).

An epidemiological study (*Indian Journal of Medical Research*, 69:776, 1979) in India compared three groups of vegetarians who consumed large amounts, small amounts, and no amount of garlic; the mean fasting cholesterol levels for these three groups were, respectively, 159, 172 and 208 milligrams per 100 milliliters of serum. The diet of all three groups was strikingly similar except for the differences in garlic and onion intake. Those who abstained completely from garlic and onions, moreover, had blood that clotted more quickly than did those who consumed garlic and onions. In another human study, Bordia (*American Journal of Clinical Nutrition*, 34:2100, 1981) compared two groups of patients with coronary-artery disease over a ten-month period. The group that received garlic supplements had steadily decreasing levels of lipoproteins associated with heart disease while in the control group, which did not receive garlic, levels of these substances remained elevated.

Garlic has been shown (*Journal of Nutrition*, 103:88, 1973) to contain certain sulfur-containing amino acids that can (*Experientia*, 30:468, 1974) interfere with the biosynthesis of fatty acids, cholesterol, triglycerides and phospholipids. More research is definitely justified.

Note on onions: Onions, which are related to garlic, have also been said to be good for the heart and circulatory system. Recently, Dr. Victor Gurewich, director of the Vascular Laboratory at St. Elizabeth's Hospital in Boston and professor of medicine at Tufts University, found that the juice of one yellow or white onion taken daily can raise high-density lipoprotein (HDL) cholesterol 30 percent in persons with abnormally low HDL. This is good because HDL, unlike other forms of cholesterol, has actually been shown to protect against cardiovascular disease. Gurewich and colleagues (according to a report in *American Health*, Nov./Dec. 1983) believe that individuals who seem to be in good health but who have abnormally low HDL levels could be at greater-than-average risk of suffering heart attacks or strokes and that daily onion juice might, therefore, help prevent these catastrophes. They are studying some two dozen onion ingredients in hope of isolating the HDL-elevating factor or factors. Gurewich thinks a combination of ingredients in raw onion juice may work together to exert an overall protective effect, so, if you like onions, indulge.

(See also discussion, later in this chapter, of capsicum—hot pepper—which also has some effects similar to those of onions and garlic.)

2) Has antibiotic effects—There are isolated reports suggesting that garlic may have some antibacterial (*Applied Microbiology*, 17:903, 1969) and antifungal (*Mycologia*, 70:397, 1978; *International Journal of Dermatology*, 19:285, 1980) effects. Here, however, a great deal more research will have to be done before anyone can justifiably claim that garlic has significant antibiotic or immunostimulant effects. Certainly the oft-heard claim that a good dose of garlic will ward off colds and flus has not, even remotely, been proved. It is interesting to note, however, that farmers in parts of Canada and elsewhere have recently begun using garlic in place of some antibiotics; these farmers have claimed that garlic is just as effective as the antibiotics (and cheaper and safer) in protecting the animals and in stimulating growth. Health officials in Canada have apparently also been impressed by the garlic preparation (made from allicin, thought to be the principal active ingredient of garlic)—so much so that they have seized supplies of it, claiming it should be classified as a drug!

3) Protects against cancer—Again, there are only a few scattered reports of garlic-related antitumor effects. (See, for example, *Cancer Research*, 18:1301, 1958; *Nature*, 216:83, 1967.) It has been reported anecdotally that high-garlic consumers in China have lower incidences of certain types of cancer than do those who use small amounts or no amount of garlic in their diet. There are also anecdotal reports that garlic applied topically helps arrest a possibly precancerous skin condition called actinic keratosis. The possibility that garlic may contain anticancer agents has been taken seriously enough that the National Cancer Institute is now requesting grant applications for the identification and study of these putative ingredients. For now, however, there is no proof that garlic is effective against cancer and no one should rely upon it as a form of treatment.

4) Increases energy—There is *one* report, based on seemingly sound data, which suggests that high doses of garlic might in-

crease physical endurance, at least in rats. Saxena and co-workers (*Indian Journal of Physiology and Pharmacology*, 24:233, 1980) were seeking to discover whether garlic might protect against drug-induced damage to heart muscle. They injected rats with the heart-damaging drug isoproterenol. One group of these rats had been given garlic supplements for seven days prior to injection with this drug; another group was given the drug too, but not the garlic. The garlic-supplemented rats withstood the effects of the drug far better than the rats that didn't get garlic. The garlic-protected rats exhibited their greater endurance by swimming 840 seconds before and 560 seconds after isoproterenol injection. The rats that did not receive garlic swam an average of 480 seconds before and only 78 seconds after injection with the drug. At autopsy, far fewer lesions were found in the heart muscles of the garlic-supplemented rats than in the myocardia of the control rats.

RELATED TO NEGATIVE CLAIMS:

1) Toxic—Garlic has low toxicity. Some individuals, however, experience gastric distress after eating garlic, especially large amounts of it. A *few* people have allergic reactions, usually manifested in the form of "contact dermatitis." This is a rash that appears after handling fresh garlic.

2) Offensive—This is a matter of individual taste—and smell. At least one researcher (*Atherosclerosis*, 44:119, 1982) has complained that the garlic dosages needed to achieve some of the favorable effects that have been reported in the medical literature are so large that many would be reluctant to take them for fear of social rejection. Perhaps a growing awareness of garlic's potential health benefits will alter our perception of garlic odor. We may even, in the future, come to think of it as the "odor of health."

IV. Recommendations

There is some evidence, cited above, that small-to-liberal amounts of garlic added to food may exert some beneficial effects on human health. My recommendation is: If you like garlic, use it, but don't use it in lieu of established remedies for specific ailments. The same applies to onions; it appears that the yellow and white ones may be more beneficial than the red ones and that raw is best.

There are a number of garlic supplements on the market. Many of these are "deodorized." The advertising claims are that the deodorized products confer all the benefits of raw or non-deodorized garlic but without the odor of garlic. These claims, however, are unproved. Lau and colleagues, cited above, note that an aging-fermentation process has been used by some of the Japanese researchers to rid garlic of some of its odor; this particular product *did* continue to exert beneficial effects (lowering cholesterol levels) in animal experiments. There is no guarantee, however, that all of the deodorizing processes will leave garlic's active ingredients intact and effective. At this point we don't even know with certainty what all those active ingredients are. It is quite possible that some of the deodorizing techniques now in use in the manufacture of garlic products may rob garlic of some of its beneficial properties. My recommendation is to stick with garlic in its natural, undeodorized form. Fresh garlic is probably the most effective.

Ginseng

I. Overview

Here's another venerable, and still somewhat inscrutable, staple of the health-food shelf. One thing is certain: This medicinal plant is neither the completely useless nor the utterly innocuous entity many believe it to be. Research to date suggests that ginseng should neither be used too casually nor should it be too easily dismissed. Of course, Chinese doctors have taken it seriously for centuries. *New Scientist* (Jan. 20, 1977, p. 138) noted that "even the Russian cosmonauts chewed ginseng as a prophylaxis against infection"; the magazine also commented on "suggestions . . . that both Henry Kissinger and Chairman Mao took it, and that it was a component of the Chinese and North Vietnamese soldiers' battle packs." It has long enjoyed a folk-medicine reputation as a general rejuvenator and life prolonger, as well as a specific protector against most of the degenerative diseases. It has attracted a cultish following for its claimed capacity to maintain and boost male sexual potency. It must be emphasized, however, that there are also studies that suggest some potentially serious pitfalls for those who use large amounts of ginseng for prolonged periods.

Ginseng, in any event, has done something important. It has called attention to the Chinese system of medicine that stresses balance, rather than antagonism, as the basic principle of healing.

II. Claims

POSITIVE:
1) Panacea/rejuvenator.

NEGATIVE:
1) Heavy use leads to the "ginseng abuse syndrome," which gives rise to elevated blood pressure, skin eruptions, diarrhea and other adverse effects; 2) may have adverse hormonal effects in both men and women.

III. Evidence

RELATED TO POSITIVE CLAIMS:

1) Panacea/rejuvenator—Ginseng is said to do everything from cure cancer to increase sexual potency and desire, so thoroughly does it stimulate and rejuvenate the entire body. Or so it is claimed. There are a number of substances in ginseng that, on the face of it, could account for some of its claimed pharmacological effects. These include peptides, sterols and saproninlike glycosides, among others, present in varying concentrations depending upon the source of the ginseng.

Perhaps the principal ginseng researcher of the world is Professor Israel Brekhman at the Soviet agency researching "biologically active substances" in Vladivostok. He and others reported (*Annual Review of Pharmacology and Toxicology*, 9:419, 1969; *Arzneimittel-Forschung/Drug Research*, 25:539, 1975) that in animal studies ginseng was capable of stimulating immune response, raising and lowering both blood sugar and blood pressure, and reducing the incidence of spontaneous mammary-gland tumors and leukemia (in mice).

Stephen Fulder, of the Department of Human Biology, Chelsea College, London, reported (see *New Scientist* article cited above) that Brekhman has also experimented with ginseng in humans, testing its effects on stamina and physical endurance among Soviet soldiers. Significant, positive results were obtained in these reportedly controlled trials, according to Fulder, who also comments on other Soviet-bloc research indicating that some properties of ginseng are active in the central nervous system. Fulder observes that this research indicates ginseng is antagonistic to depressants such as alcohol and barbiturates and that it is often a mood elevator. The stimulant effects of ginseng in some individuals have been confirmed in a two-year study by Siegel (*Journal of the American Medical Association*, 241:1641, 1979), who also, however, noted several adverse side effects (see below).

Claims that ginseng can increase male sexual potency are persistent and widespread but remain purely anecdotal. Interestingly, there have also been some isolated anecdotal claims that prolonged usage of ginseng can have masculinizing effects in some women. One woman claimed to have grown a highly visible moustache that receded after she discontinued using ginseng. And there have been a few undocumented reports of women developing the so-called "dowager's hump," a hunchbacked condition caused by bone deformity that characterizes some postmenopausal women who do not receive estrogen-replacement therapy.

"It is probable," Fulder writes, "that the rich mixture of glycosides and other constituents within the plant results in apparently paradoxical effects. Indeed, Japanese workers have shown that one isolated and characterized terpenoidal glycoside can be stimulatory while another depressant."

Ginseng is an intriguing substance worthy of further research. Until that research is carried out, however, we have no way of knowing much about either its long-term safety or efficacy.

RELATED TO NEGATIVE CLAIMS:

1) Heavy use leads to the "ginseng abuse syndrome," which gives rise to elevated blood pressure, skin eruptions, diarrhea and other adverse effects—This is the syndrome identified by Siegel (cited above), who studied 133 users of ginseng over a period of two years. He noted various stimulatory and euphoric effects in some of these subjects but also observed a pattern of

adverse effects, including morning diarrhea (experienced by 47 of the 133 subjects), skin eruptions (33 subjects), sleeplessness (26 subjects), nervousness (25 subjects), high blood pressure (22 subjects) and edema—swelling of tissues—(14 subjects). Those studied ingested varying amounts of ginseng from numerous sources, including teas, roots, tablets, and even intranasal and injectable preparations.

The "ginseng abuse syndrome" was defined as elevated blood pressure combined with nervousness, insomnia, skin eruptions and morning diarrhea. The full syndrome was experienced by fourteen subjects who took approximately 3 grams of oral ginseng daily. One subject exhibited notable withdrawal symptoms when ginseng was abruptly discontinued; these symptoms included hypotension (abnormally low blood pressure), weakness and tremor. It should be noted, however, that this study was not controlled, and several of the subjects (though by no means all of those who experienced adverse effects) were also using some other drugs in addition to ginseng.

2) May have adverse hormonal effects in both men and women —There have been anecdotal reports that heavy ginseng intake can have masculinizing effects in women and feminizing effects in men (such as enlargement of breasts). Palmer et al. reported (*British Medical Journal*, 1:1284, 1978) that a seventy-year-old woman experienced tenderness, swelling and diffuse nodularity of the breasts on three occasions after taking ginseng. There have been other such reports (*British Medical Journal*, 1:1556, 1978). A 1980 report (*British Medical Journal*, 281:1110, 1980) noted an apparent estrogenic effect on the epithelium of the vagina in a sixty-two-year-old woman; the effect was related to ginseng intake. These reports, though uncontrolled, lend further credibility to the precaution that ginseng is a pharmacologically active substance that should not be used casually.

IV. Recommendations

Pending the outcome of future studies, I do not recommend that ginseng be used in any form for any reason. Be particularly cautious about using ginseng "extracts," inhalants, capsules, tablets and roots. If you must take ginseng, stick to the teas, though I don't recommend them either. Many people drink these teas without any apparent ill effects and so assume that other, more concentrated forms of ginseng will be similarly innocuous. As some of the research cited above indicates, this may not be true. And what is innocuous in one person may produce an adverse effect in another. Ginseng is a very interesting substance that deserves further research. Until that research is done, the prudent consumer will make no assumptions as to either the safety or the efficacy of ginseng.

Pangamic Acid ("Vitamin B-15")

I. Overview

Here's a can of worms. Discovered by the same folks who developed "laetrile," pangamic acid, or "vitamin B_{15}," as it is popularly, but erroneously, known, has been a best seller every year since 1978. It was that year that *New York* magazine (Mar. 13, 1978) screamed across its cover: "WONDER DRUG B_{15} cures alcoholism, hepatitis, heart disease, allergies, diabetes, schizophrenia, glaucoma, keeps you young, and purifies the very air you breathe." Apparently out of breath themselves, the editors then paused long enough to add one word: "Maybe." The article itself proceeded in the same—let's have it both ways—spirit, basically touting B_{15} to the heavens while occasionally slipping in some mild disclaimer. Everybody from Muhammad Ali to Dick Gregory was said to be popping the stuff, which was supposed to have been discovered in the pits of apricots.

There was scarcely anything B_{15} wasn't capable of, according to the various sources quoted by *New York*. Its credentials as a panacea were said to be based on its extreme potency as an "oxygenator" of body tissues, bringing them all up to optimal snuff, enhancing, among other things, the "brilliance" and "flash" of orgasm, increasing one's ability to do yoga, mopping up free radicals like mad, saving people from the need for amputation of gangrenous limbs, etc., etc. In no time, of course, nearly every health-food/vitamin store in the country had banners in their windows proclaiming: "B_{15} sold here!" People are still buying.

It would be wonderful if pangamic acid (which is not a vitamin by any stretch of the imagination; there is no evidence whatever that the body has any dietary need of it) could do even a small fraction of the things claimed for it. Unfortunately, there is only scant evidence that it can have any therapeutic effect in *any* ailment. And even then the prospects for the consumer are bleak because product mislabeling is rampant. Worse —if proved—are recent claims that two of the major ingredients of several of the B_{15} products still being marketed are potential carcinogens.

II. Claims

POSITIVE:
1) Tissue oxygenator, panacea and general "miracle" substance.

NEGATIVE:
1) Cancer-causing.

III. Evidence

RELATED TO POSITIVE CLAIMS:

1) Tissue oxygenator, panacea and general "miracle" substance —Almost all of the claims made for pangamic acid or dimethylglycine (DMG), which is the hypothesized active ingredient, are based upon Soviet research. Stacpoole, in a review (*World Review of Nutrition and Dietetics*, 27:145, 1977) of the largely Russian research, noted that "nearly all of these studies suffer from methodologic flaws which seriously limit their probative value. Often, patient populations and diagnostic criteria are incompletely described, and comparisons between treated subjects and suitably matched controls are lacking." McCarty (*Medical Hypotheses*, 7:515, 1981) has similarly faulted the Soviet research, noting "the methodological laxness and wild-eyed enthusiasm of Russian clinical reports." Claims that DMG has lipotropic effects (promoting optimal utilization of fats) are persistent in the literature and are not in themselves farfetched, but, as McCarty adds, "there is no indication that [DMG] is more efficacious in this regard than cheaper and less exotic factors such as choline. . . ."

Studies of DMG outside the Soviet Union have generally failed to find any therapeutic value in it. Roach and Gibson (*Annals of Neurology*, 14:347, 1983) recently reported that DMG is of no value in the treatment of epileptic patients with refractory seizures (the type that do not yield to standard medications). Their study was double-blind. Grabner and co-workers (*Journal of Infectious Diseases*, 143:101, 1981), in a double-blind study of 20 human volunteers, report a significant DMG-induced enhancement of both humoral- and cell-mediated immune response, but there is no confirmation of this work.

It is unfortunate that there has been so much hype and so many unsubstantiated claims made for DMG. It is possible that it may have some positive value, but most researchers are now loath to investigate DMG for fear of fueling even higher hopes for the substance. This fear is heightened by the possibility that DMG may have harmful side effects (see below).

RELATED TO NEGATIVE CLAIMS:

1) Cancer-causing—There is evidence that DMG, thought by many to be the active product of pangamic acid, may be mutagenic and thus potentially able to cause cancer. In the widely accepted test of mutagenesis (reported upon in the *Journal of the American Medical Association*, 243:2473, 1980), substances that turn out to be mutagenic have, according to one survey, a 90 percent probability of being carcinogenic as well. Neville Colman, M.D., of the Hematology and Nutrition Laboratory of the Bronx Veterans Administration Medical Center in New York, "concluded," according to the *JAMA* article cited above, "that the main component of this vitamin B_{15} formulation is capable of reacting to form a potential carcinogen under conditions simulating those found in the human digestive tract." Gerlernt and Herbert (*Nutrition and Cancer*, 3:129, 1982) report that diisopropylamine-dichloracetate (DIPA-DCA), the major constituent of another best-selling pangamic product, is also mutagenic. These findings, though they require confirmation by others, constitute ominous red flags.

The FDA has sought to have pangamic acid banned as an unsafe food additive. Pangamic acid may, indeed, be unsafe, but the additive argument may be doomed since it can be demonstrated that DMG, at least, is an intermediary metabolite naturally present in many foods. In any event, the intelligent consumer will steer clear of any and all products said to be "pangamic acid," "calcium pangamate," "B_{15}" or anything related thereto. Apart from the possibility of carcinogenicity, consumers are herewith warned that analyses of products on the market at the present time make it evident that no one can have any confidence that these products contain what's on the label.

IV. Recommendations

My recommendation is unequivocal: *Don't* use any products labeled or related to "pangamic acid," "calcium pangamate" or "B$_{15}$," Product mislabeling is rampant, and some of the substances included in these products may be carcinogens. (See discussion above under Related to Negative Claims.)

Superoxide Dismutase (SOD)

I. Overview

"Superoxide Dismutase—Field Marshal in the Battle with Age!" So reads the headline of an unattributed promotional handout available in many health-food/vitamin stores. Superoxide dismutase (SOD) is being widely touted as the super antioxidant of all time, the "hero" supplement that will "save" our cells from the relentless savagery of the free radicals. In the process of extending our life-spans, SOD, it is claimed, will also rescue us from arthritis, cancer and even the side effects of radiation.

All true? Unfortunately, no. SOD is an enzyme that, in its different forms, is associated with copper, zinc and manganese. There is good evidence that SOD is, indeed, an antioxidant that helps protect cells against some of the adverse effects of oxidant damage (see Chapter One). SOD *does* show promise as a therapeutic agent, but *not* in the form being sold in the vitamin stores. Oral SOD, as explained in more detail below, is destroyed in the gut before it can reach the blood. Oral supplements are worthless rip-offs. The aggressive marketing of oral-SOD products by a number of companies is an example of the sort of abuse that has made it possible for many physicians to dismiss nutritional supplements, as a whole, out of hand. The damage done in this respect is even more harmful than that done to the trusting consumer who buys a worthless product.

II. Claims

POSITIVE:
1) Retards aging; 2) protects against arthritis; 3) protects against cancer; 4) protects against radiation damage.

NEGATIVE:
1) Worthless in oral form.

III. Evidence

RELATED TO POSITIVE CLAIMS:

1) Retards aging—"The fountain of youth can be yours—in one easy-to-take pill form," proclaims the *National Enquirer*, July 28, 1981. Some of the makers of SOD products have made similar claims—all without foundation. There is no evidence whatever that SOD supplements can retard aging.

2) Protects against arthritis—This claim derives from research (see discussion of same under Evidence: Related to Positive Claims in the analysis of copper earlier in this book) in which *injections* of bovine copper-zinc SOD (known as Orgotein) showed some promise as an anti-inflammatory agent in osteoarthritis and rheumatoid arthritis. There is no evidence whatever that oral SOD has similar effects. As explained under Related to Negative Claims below, there is, in fact, no reason to believe that it would or could.

3) Protects against cancer—Michelson and collaborators have reported (*Superoxide and Superoxide Dismutases*, Academic Press, New York, 1977, p. 496) increased survival times in SOD-treated hamsters with transplanted melanoma tumors. But, again, the SOD used was of the injectable variety. In any event, much more research will have to be done before SOD in any form can be said to have confirmed anticancer properties. Such research is warranted.

4) Protects against radiation damage—Michelson and co-workers (cited above) report that some of the adverse side effects of radiation can be diminished via SOD *injections*. Extrapolating

from these findings, which, though based on sound methodology, require confirmation, various SOD enthusiasts have claimed that the oral-SOD preparations being sold in vitamin stores can similarly protect against radiation. One widely distributed health-food handout declares that "SOD should be in everybody's cabinet as a first-aid measure against nuclear-plant accidents as well as accidents in transporting nuclear wastes." This crock of cranberries apparently originates with Passwater (*Selenium as Food and Medicine*, Keats Publishing, Hartford, Conn., 1980, pp. 96–99), who recommends that "your radiation defense first-aid kit should include kelp or potassium iodine tablets, superoxide dismutase tablets and antioxidants. . . ." Save your money. I'm appalled that people are out there pushing worthless oral-SOD products, horrified that they are using radiation scare tactics to help sell this junk.

RELATED TO NEGATIVE CLAIMS:

1) Worthless in oral form—This claim has been substantiated. Zidenberg-Cherr and co-workers (*American Journal of Clinical Nutrition*, 37:5, 1983) convincingly demonstrated that oral SOD is digested in the gut before it can be absorbed by the blood and delivered to target tissues. There is *no* oral SOD on the market today that evades this problem; nor is there every likely to be in the future. Injectable SOD, which is still experimental and requires close medical supervision, *does* evade destruction in the gut and so has at least the *potential* of having therapeutic value in certain disorders, as outlined above.

IV. Recommendations

For reasons explained above, do *not* buy or use *any* of the oral-SOD products on the market. They are entirely worthless.

Wheatgrass/Barley Grass (And Some Other Green Plants)

I. Overview

Wheatgrass and barley grass, either as juices or as sprouts, are being promoted increasingly as "wonder" substances. Health-food/vitamin stores across the nation are selling them with claims that they confer protection against a variety of pollutants and even against radiation. They are said to detoxify the body, purify the blood and protect against cancer. These claims have until very recently been based almost entirely upon anecdotal testimonials. Happily, it turns out that there may be *some* substance to at least some of these alleged benefits.

"Eat-Die," "Eat-Die," "Eat-Die." That pessimistic prescription was written over and over across the cover of *Science* magazine. It related to an article written by the noted biochemist Bruce Ames, who reported (*Science*, 221:1256, 1983) on the increasing number of cancer-causing substances being found in the food we routinely eat. Fortunately, there is some good news, as well. We are beginning to find that some of the foods we eat —or should eat—may also protect against cancer. Certain green plants and vegetables may be among these.

II. Claims

POSITIVE:
1) Slows aging and fights cancer.

III. Evidence

RELATED TO POSITIVE CLAIMS:

1) Slows aging and fights cancer—Lai et al. (*Nutrition and Cancer*, 1:27, 1978) found that extracts from the roots and leaves of wheat sprouts selectively inhibited the mutagenic effect of carcinogens in the Ames Test (commonly used to determine cancer-causing potential of substances under study). Chlorophyll, the pigment that gives plants their green color and is fundamental for the conversion of the sun's energy into carbohydrates, has been identified as one of the factors that inhibit the mutagenic effect of carcinogens requiring metabolic activation (*Nutrition and Cancer*, 1:19, 1979). Chlorophyll is capable of electron transfer (see Chapter One) and may indeed function as an antioxidant.

The biologist Yasuo Hotta (personal communication) is doing some promising work with an extract of lyophilized (freeze-dried) barley grass (similar to wheatgrass). He finds (reported at the Annual Meeting of Japan Pharmaceutical Sciences, Apr. 3, 1982, Osaka) that this extract protects human fibroblasts and lung cells grown in tissue culture against cell damage from X rays and a cancer-causing agent, 4-nitroso-quinoline. The extract must be given to the cells *before* the damaging agent is introduced for this protective function to occur. Chlorophyll does not appear to be the active factor in this case.

Hotta (reported at the Annual Meeting of Japan Pharmaceutical Sciences, Apr. 15, 1982, Kumamato) also finds that germ cells of older mice are protected against damage to their DNA during one phase of cell division by an extract of barley grass. The phase in question is one in which the DNA is particularly vulnerable to damage. Vulnerability seems to increase with age. Again, chlorophyll does not seem to be the active protective agent. Hotta has identified a substance from barley grass that *does* seem to be one of the active characters; it seems to have superoxide-dismutase-like activity. It is anticipated that further research will shed light on its nature and function.

This exciting new research recalls some much earlier, now largely forgotten work. Lourau and Lartigue (*Experientia*, 6:25, 1950) studied some of the effects diet can have on the body's response to X-radiation. They noted that guinea pigs exposed to whole-body X-radiation had lower mortality and incidence of hemorrhage when prefed on cabbage than when prefed on beets. This study shows how dramatically times have changed. Rather than conclude that there could be something *protective* against radiation in cabbage, these researchers chose to account for the differences observed by assuming that there was something in beets that became highly toxic in irradiated animals. The idea that something in food could be a significant protector against something like radiation was just too unheard of at that time to take seriously.

Some time later, however, spurred by the intriguing experiment of Lourau and Lartigue, Spector and Calloway (*Proceedings of the Society for Experimental Biology and Medicine*, 100:405, 1959) decided to investigate further. They again exposed guinea pigs to whole-body X-radiation after first having fed them for two weeks on varying diets. *All* of the control animals fed on rations of oats and wheat bran died within fifteen days of irradiation. Experimental animals that received the oats and wheat bran *supplemented with raw cabbage* had in seven separate trials an average reduced mortality of 52 percent. Another member of the cabbage family—broccoli—was found, in an additional two trials, to be even more protective against radiation damage. In still more trials, both pre- and postirradiation feeding of cabbage was found to exert statistically significant protective effects, but the most positive effects were achieved when cabbage was given both before and after irradiation.

Now, more than three decades after the initial report of Lourau and Lartigue and some twenty-five years after the work of Spector and Calloway, there is renewed interest in the possible anticancer properties of some green plants. Dr. Frank J. Rauscher, Jr., the American Cancer Society's vice-president for research, told those gathered at the Annual Meeting of the society's Illinois division in September 1983 that new research (at the University of Minnesota) has shown that there is something in Brussels sprouts (*another* member of the cabbage family) that inhibits the development of certain cancers in laboratory animals. Two substances have been isolated and are under study.

The cancer work of Hotta and others is intriguing and should be encouraged.

IV. Recommendations

There is no hard evidence at hand at the present time that proves that barley grass, wheatgrass, plants in the cabbage family and so on inhibit cancers in humans. There are data suggestive of cancer-protecting effects in some animals. More research is certainly warranted. In the meantime, it appears that no harm can come of eating these green plants. If you like them, by all means, indulge. They contain vitamins and minerals—and *possibly* something more.

Miscellaneous Supplements

The following "other supplements" are treated in less formal fashion than the foregoing, either because research is largely lacking or because some of the substances discussed are only now emerging in the marketplace. Some are already best sellers, propelled, in some instances, by advertising and promotional hype and, in others, by genuinely satisfied word-of-mouth or persistent folklore.

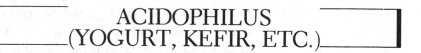

ACIDOPHILUS (YOGURT, KEFIR, ETC.)

Yogurt, kefir and some other health-food items are milk fermented by the bacterium *Lactobacillus acidophilus* (and other bacteria). Acidophilus and various of its products are said, without documentation, to lower cholesterol levels, clear the skin, extend life-span, enhance immunity, etc. Acidophilus *is* useful in the maintenance of intestinal and vaginal ecological balance. People taking oral antibiotics (including women taking vaginal antibiotics) over long periods of time may benefit from oral acidophilus or intravaginal acidophilus. Acidophilus helps keep alive those harmless or useful microorganisms that if eliminated might be replaced by potentially harmful pathogens. Many doctors recommend acidophilus for the purpose of preventing, for example, yeast infections of the vagina. (Do not use acidophilus intravaginally, however, without directions to do so from your doctor.) There are many anecdotal reports that people feel better, in general, when they regularly consume products that contain acidophilus. The often-heard claims that cultures (no pun intended) in which yogurt is a primary staple of daily diet produce an excessive number of happy ancients are unproved. There is no reason, however, to discourage the consumption of these products. A recent report shows yogurt to be a well-tolerated source of milk for lactase-deficient persons (*New England Journal of Medicine*, 310:1, 1984).

ALOE VERA

Aloe vera has been widely proclaimed (in the health-food literature) as "the miracle plant." The juices and gels of this yucca-like plant have become big sellers in recent years. Even *Runner's World* (Jan. 1983) ran an article called "Aloe Vera and Athletes: The Miracle Plant Helps the Athlete Stay Healthy." Claims that aloe vera helps burns heal more quickly, that it's good for the skin, that it relieves the pain and speeds the repair of athletic injuries, that it is a diet aid, an anticancer substance, a cure for ulcers, an antifungal agent, even a remedy for bed-wetting, all remain purely anecdotal. Some of these anecdotes have persisted for centuries, during which time aloe vera has been used as a folk remedy for numerous ills in many different cultures. There are a number of ingredients in aloe vera, including minerals and vitamins, amino acids, enzymes and a salicylatelike substance that, hypothetically, could help reduce inflammation and pain associated with burns (see R. Ruldoph and J. Noe, *Chronic Problem Wounds*, Little, Brown, Boston, 1983). There's probably no harm in trying aloe vera as a *topical* ointment for mild burns and mosquito bites, but don't look for "miraculous" results. And do *not* believe claims that aloe vera can do anything to prevent or treat cancer. There is no evidence whatever that this is true.

BEE POLLEN

Bee pollen has been called "nature's most perfect food." The therapeutic claims made for bee pollen have been similarly immodest. It's supposed to energize the body, regulate the bowels, dispel prostate problems, regulate weight, renew the skin, ward off heart disease and arthritis, relieve stress, boost immunity, inhibit cancer, diminish allergies and so on—and on. A number of "notables," including Ronald Reagan, have been known to indulge in bee pollen, according to press reports, many of which also claim that bee pollen is an all-around anti-aging agent of the first water. Some pollen promoters concede that there is no scientific evidence to support any of these claims; but neither, they add, are there any to debunk them. Some others claim the Soviets are working feverishly to unlock the many "secrets" of bee pollen. One pollen enthusiast went so far as to speak of "an actual bee-pollen knowledge gap between our two countries." In fact, however, there is no reliable research, in either the U.S. or the Soviet Union, that suggests you can benefit in any way from bee pollen. Something might eventually turn up, but for now bee pollen is a very expensive way of getting inadequate and uncertain supplies of a few vitamins, minerals and amino acids. The "pollen power" that promoters like to talk about is all at the cash register.

BIOFLAVONOIDS

Here is a riches-to-rags story. Found in considerable quantities in most fruits and vegetables and especially in citrus fruits, the bioflavonoids were once widely prescribed by physicians under the lofty label of "vitamin P," so named by the distinguished Hungarian researcher Albert Szent-Gyorgyi, who won the Nobel Prize in Medicine for, among other things, his discovery of vitamin C. It was in the course of isolating vitamin C that Szent-Gyorgyi came across the bioflavonoids. He had a friend with bleeding gums and thought this condition might have something to do with a vitamin C deficiency. He gave the man some of his early, impure vitamin C preparation and, sure enough, the man's bleeding gums cleared up.

Later on, confronted by a recurrence of the bleeding gums, Szent-Gyorgyi decided to try again—this time with his newly purified vitamin C. He expected to observe an even more dramatic result this second time. No such luck. The man's gums went right on bleeding. Szent-Gyorgyi re-examined his earlier preparation and decided that the effective impurity was one of the bioflavonoids. He tried those—by themselves—and reported that they worked (for a review of the bioflavonoid literature, see *The Anti-Inflammatory Action of Flavonoids* by Miklos Gabor, with a foreword by Albert Szent-Gyorgyi, Akademiai Kiado, Budapest, 1972). The bioflavonoids thus came into use primarily as protectors of capillaries, the tiniest blood vessels in the body. The bioflavonoids were said to strengthen or preserve the structural integrity of these vessels, preventing bleeding disorders related to numerous maladies.

Thousands of doctors in the U.S. began prescribing bioflavonoids, encouraged by dozens of studies that showed their efficacy. Then, in 1968, the Food and Drug Administration, relying primarily upon a review of the bioflavonoid literature conducted by a panel of the National Academy of Sciences/National Research Council, withdrew the bioflavonoid drugs from the marketplace, declaring that they were ineffective in humans "for any condition" whatsoever. The more than fifty drug companies, including many of the pharmaceutical giants, that had been manufacturing bioflavonoid preparations for prescription use were obliged to halt production—at least for distribution in the U.S.

Overall, this was a curious episode. The *Medical Letter,* in an article called "Requiem for Flavonoid Drugs," Feb. 9, 1968, p. 9, voiced its support for the FDA action but acknowledged that "many of the authors who investigated these drugs and found them effective were as competent as most of the authors whose reports on drugs now appear in medical journals, and their studies were of about the same quality as many of the studies now being reported." The *Medical Letter* was trying to say that even competent researchers make mistakes. True enough. But, looking back, one has to wonder if the dozens of independent researchers whose findings tended to confirm one another shouldn't be considered more trustworthy than the conclusions of a single review panel. Review panels also make mistakes.

Szent-Gyorgyi, right or wrong, concluded that the FDA action was largely political. He noted that there had always been resistance among some in the American medical establishment to his designation of the bioflavonoids as a vitamin. Here was an "upstart" substance that was getting too much attention and very possibly being overprescribed in some areas. But, in addition, Szent-Gyorgyi noted, most Americans get more than enough bioflavonoids in their daily diets. Hence there was (and is) no genuine bioflavonoid deficiency in the U.S. and thus scant indication for the use of these substances in this country. This was not so, Szent-Gyorgyi argued, in many other countries where flavonoid-rich citrus fruits were in short supply and/or were too expensive for many people to buy.

Whatever the case, it is interesting to look back at some of the pre-1968 reports in respected journals observing favorable bioflavonoid effects. Here, for example, is the conclusion of a report in the *American Journal of Obstetrics and Gynecology,* 83:1269, 1962: "Oral-treatment with water-soluble citrus bioflavonoids and ascorbic acid causes a marked reduction in the blood loss of most women with regular ovulatory menorrhagia [mid-cycle bleeding] . . . menorrhagia has been shown to return in 4 to 6 weeks if control capsules [placebos] are substituted and to improve again with renewed treatment . . . both the capillary strength and the blood losses were measured objectively. . . ." Here is the conclusion of a report in the *Annals of the New York Academy of Science*, 61:732, 1955): "Taking everything together, there can be little doubt that flavonoids are not only useful therapeutic agents in conditions of capillary fragility, but have many diverse actions in the animal body."

The 1968 FDA directive prevented physicians from prescribing bioflavonoids but did nothing to prevent the consumer from purchasing them at almost any vitamin store. They go on selling in large quantities today—often teamed with vitamin C. The claim is made that vitamin C cannot be fully or properly utilized by the human body except in the presence of bioflavonoids. This—rather than the old claims concerning capillary protection—is why most consumers purchase bioflavonoids today. Ironically, it is *this* claim that certainly does not hold water. It is based on early findings (*Nature*, 161:557, 1948) that bioflavonoids increase the utilization of ascorbic acid (vitamin C) *in guinea pigs*. Pelletier and Keith, however, showed (*Journal of the American Dietetic Association*, 64:271, 1974) that this does not hold true in man. They found, in fact, that *synthetic* vitamin C is more "bioavailable," i.e., is better absorbed and utilized by the human body, than either ascorbic acid teamed with rutin (a widely sold bioflavonoid) or "natural" vitamin C in the form of orange juice!

"It is not surprising," these researchers concluded, "that bioflavonoids affect ascorbic acid utilization differently in man than in guinea pigs. In guinea pigs, ascorbic acid is rapidly broken down to carbon dioxide, producing a half-life of ascorbic acid of four days compared with eighteen days in man. The protection against oxidation afforded ascorbic acid by bioflavonoids should be more important for guinea pigs than man."

Vitamin C products that come "fortified" with or "protected" by bioflavonoids tend to be considerably more expensive than vitamin C alone. Save your money. The claim that bioflavonoids are needed for full utilization of vitamin C is contradicted by the best available evidence. As for claims that bioflavonoids protect the capillaries, that matter, while perhaps deserving of re-examination, remains unsettled; in any event, however, the data related thereto are thought to apply only to individuals with genuine flavonoid *deficiencies*. As even the discoverer of the bioflavonoids has pointed out, it is likely that such deficiencies are extremely rare in the U.S.

BREWER'S YEAST

Just about every ailment you can imagine is supposed to be subject to the mysterious powers of brewer's yeast. *One* of the problems with this claim is that the nutritional values of yeasts can vary tremendously. Yeast *can* be a good source of many B vitamins and of protein, but quality and quantity of nutrients in yeast are, from the consumer's point of view, generally unpredictable. Specific therapeutic claims for brewer's yeast have not been substantiated. (See, however, my analysis of chromium for a discussion of the better-established benefits of chromium-enriched yeast and glucose tolerance factor.)

CAPSICUM (HOT PEPPER)

Capsicum (hot pepper) has long been used by some as a reputed tonic for gastric and intestinal problems and as a pain-killer for toothache. Others claim capsicum can ward off infections and promote overall good health. Most such claims are anecdotal, but in 1982 a group of researchers in Thailand reported (*American Journal of Clinical Nutrition*, 35:1452, 1982) that the daily ingestion of capsicum by most of the Thai people, who use the hot pepper as a seasoning and an appetizer, may be associated with the low incidence of thromboembolic (potentially fatal blood clotting) diseases in that country. The researchers found that capsicum has a definite fibrinolytic activity, meaning that it can, to some degree, break down clots through an enzymatic mechanism. Significantly greater fibrinolytic activity was detected in Thais who consume capsicum several times a day than among Americans living in Thailand who consumed primarily American-style meals and little or no capsicum.

While the Thai researchers concede that theirs is a preliminary study, they note that the fibrinolytic activation they observed was possibly "sufficient to prevent thromboembolism among the majority of such [regular] consumers" of capsicum. And they add: "More investigations on this effect may lead to the discovery of some ideal drugs for both treatment and prevention of thromboembolism." They cite other research attributing lesser but still measurable fibrinolytic activity to the regular intake of onions, chilies and various hot spices. They also note that there is a low incidence of thromboembolism not only among the Thais but also among the New Guineans, East Africans, South African Bantus, Nigerians, Melanesians, Koreans and Indians. Most, if not all, of these peoples are known for favoring hot and spicy foods.

Given the high incidence of thromboembolism in many parts of the world, including the U.S., this preliminary research has to be accounted interesting and worthy of follow-up.

Another claim made for capsicum is that it can be used to treat toothache. A drop or two of hot-pepper extract applied on cotton to the aching tooth was recommended by the Dublin medical press in 1950, claiming that the hot pepper would quell the pain. There appears to be some support for this idea (*Lancet*, 1:1198, 1983).

If you are thinking of adding capsicum, which has been available in health-food stores for years, to your daily diet, do so in moderation. The Thai research indicates it doesn't take much hot pepper—used primarily as a seasoning—to produce a fibrinolytic effect. And the consumer should be aware that I am talking about *red* hot pepper. Black pepper appears to have a carcinogenic principle, at least in mice (*Science*, 221:1256, 1983), and does *not* have the fibrinolytic effect that red pepper does. People taking anticoagulants should use hot-pepper and capsicum preparations with caution—so as not to overdo. If your doctor has prescribed anticoagulants or you have a problem with bleeding (slow clotting time), check with a physician before making capsicum a part of your regular diet. Also be aware that a few people report that hot pepper upsets—rather than settles —their stomachs. If you are one of those people you should not use hot pepper.

CHONDROITIN SULFATE

Chondroitin sulfate is a substance found in the cartilages of most mammals, including man. Research interest in this substance has increased in recent years and you are bound to be hearing more about it in the future. Claims made for it have been related primarily to various forms of heart and bone disease. In one study (*Journal of International Medical Research*, 6:217, 1978) of 46 elderly patients with narrowing of the arteries, there was evidence that chondroitin sulfate could lower cholesterol and triglyceride concentrations in the blood and prolong clotting times (a potential protective factor against dangerous clots). Further research is needed. The use of chondroitin sulfate as a food supplement is still premature and not recommended at this time.

COENZYME Q

Coenzyme Q is almost certain to be touted soon as one of the "hottest" new supplements around. It is part of the system across which electrons flow in the mitochondria of cells (see Chapter One) in the process of energy production and, as such, is biologically very important. Folkers (*American Journal of Clinical Nutrition*, 27:1026, 1974) has shown the relationship of coenzyme Q and vitamin E, which, nonetheless, have many distinct functions. Folkers and co-workers (*Journal of Molecular Medicine*, 2:431, 1977) have reviewed a decade of coenzyme Q research that, among other things, has demonstrated that CoQ "has the nutritional nature of a vitamin, but is unique in that it is not only present in many food stuffs of man's diet, but it is also biosynthesized within mammalian tissue." Deficiency states may occur.

Preliminary studies suggest that CoQ may have a number of potentially valuable therapeutic actions, but most of the interest to date has focused on its possible impact on cardiovascular disease. Some of these studies have detected CoQ-induced improvement of heart-muscle metabolism and effectiveness in the treatment of coronary insufficiency and congestive heart failure (see Folkers cited above).

Recently, researchers at the Methodist Hospital in Indianapolis and at the Institute for Bio-Medical Research at the University of Texas announced that they are treating heart-failure patients with CoQ (see report in *Resident and Staff Physician*, 29:102, 1983) with considerable success. CoQ is said by these researchers to enhance the pumping capacity of the heart and to eliminate the often major side effects associated with conventional heart-failure drugs. Heart-failure patients were said to have a relative deficiency of CoQ in their hearts and to be responsive to daily oral supplements of CoQ, which, it is reported, increases the production of energy in heart-muscle cells. Some 91 percent of the patients studied showed improvement within thirty days of beginning CoQ supplementation. Certainly more investigation of this intriguing vitaminlike nutrient is warranted. For now, however, it would be premature to recommend the use of CoQ as a dietary supplement.

GLANDULARS

"Raw glandular concentrates"—usually referred to simply as "glandulars"—are being marketed by an increasing number of companies. This isn't a revival of the old "monkey-gland operation," but it's equally as ridiculous. The simpleminded argument is that aging is largely a function of failing glands; ergo, those glands can be revived and rejuvenated, at least to some extent, by eating the concentrates of various animal glands. Claims are made that glandulars can reverse everything from hypoglycemia to cancer. Glandulars are supposed to be particularly useful in propping up sagging sex drives. One company has even put out his-and-her glandular formulas for more effective sexual functioning. Some body-builders have also begun taking glandulars, buying claims that they can help build muscle. There is *no* convincing, legitimate evidence whatever that any of these claims has any substance. Nor is there any biochemical reason to even suspect that these substances would be useful. Some of them, in fact, may be harmful; it is possible that some of these organ concentrates contain some of the many toxins livestock are exposed to, such as antibiotics, growth hormones, pesticides, herbicides, fertilizers, etc. There are often higher concentrations of these toxins in the organs than in the other tissues of these animals. Avoid glandulars.

PABA

There's one undisputed positive use for PABA (para-aminoben-zoic acid)—as a topical sunscreen to shield the skin from the damage of ultraviolet radiation. Beyond this the claims for PABA, as a skin rejuvenator and anti-arthritis substance, are anecdotal. Other anecdotal claims persist that supplemental PABA can halt hair loss and restore color to graying or white hair, but you can also talk to many who have tried PABA for these purposes without success. I do not recommend PABA except as a topical sunscreen. Those who do take it should be aware that it causes nausea and diarrhea in some individuals. In addition, PABA is stored in the tissues and in continued high dosage may prove toxic to the liver. Some enthusiasts have rec-ommended daily doses of a gram or higher; these could prove perilous. If for some reason you feel compelled to take PABA internally, do not take more than 30 milligrams daily in supple-mental form. (Natural sources of PABA include liver, kidney, whole grains, wheat germ, brown rice, bran.) Do not take PABA if you are using any of the "sulfa drugs" (sulfonamide antibiot-ics); PABA will seriously diminish their effectiveness. (See anal-ysis of Gerovital H3, next chapter, for more on PABA.)

ROYAL JELLY

Royal jelly is a "miracle substance" for at least one entity—the queen bee. This milky-white gelatinous substance is secreted in the salivary glands of worker bees for the sole apparent purpose of stimulating the growth and development of queen bees. What it can do for humans is a far more controversial matter. The claims are exuberant; it's supposed to extend life-span and, in general, reinvigorate the body. Royal jelly is rich in pantothenic acid (part of the vitamin B complex; see analysis of pantothenic acid earlier in this book), a substance essential for many meta-bolic processes.

Pantothenic acid, as previously discussed, has shown some evidence of being useful in the treatment of some bone and joint disorders. Barton-Wright and Elliot (*Lancet*, 2:862, 1963) reported that relief from various of the symptoms of rheumatoid arthritis could be achieved with injections of pantothenic acid. Intriguingly, even better results were reported by these researchers when pantothenic acid was combined with royal jelly, suggesting there might be some additional therapeutic agent in the latter. Daily intramuscular injections of royal jelly alone proved ineffective, but daily injections of a mixture of royal jelly and pantothenic acid resulted in greater improvement than had been noted with pantothenic acid alone.

Barton-Wright and Elliot hypothesized that the possible additional therapeutic factor in royal jelly might be a substance called 10-hydroxydec-2-enoic acid, as this is another major constituent of the jelly. These researchers noted in passing that Townsend and co-workers had reported earlier (*Nature*, 183:1270, 1959) that "the injection of royal jelly or of 10-hydroxydec-2-enoic acid . . . affords complete protection against transplantable mouse leukemia." I know of no follow-up to this finding, but in 1980 the General Practitioner Research Group became the first to re-examine and then confirm some of the findings of Barton Wright and Elliot with respect to calcium pantothenate (pantothenic acid) and various arthritic conditions. *Martindale—The Extra Pharmacopeia* (The Pharmaceutical Press, London, 1982, p. 1752) notes that 10-hydroxydec-2-enoic acid "has anti-microbial properties."

At this point I cannot say that people who are spending their money on royal jelly have bees in their collective bonnets. Neither, however, can I recommend the stuff, though I *do* recommend pantothenic acid, as outlined in my analysis of that substance. More research on royal jelly is needed and deserved.

SPIRULINA

Spirulina was one of those overnight sensations in the food-supplement marketplace a few years ago and is still going strong, despite the fact that it is expensive and tastes terrible. It is prepared from a blue-green alga. It is supposed to be a diet aid, good for the skin, and a general tonic and rejuvenator—in short, another panacea. There's nothing in the scientific literature to support the claims made for spirulina, save for one report which only notes (*Lipids*, 3:46, 1968) that this alga is rich in gamma-linolenic acid (GLA), the same substance that is being derived today, for the most part, from oil of evening primrose. Oil of evening primrose/GLA is one of the rising stars of the supplement marketplace (see previous analysis). How good a source of GLA spirulina really is remains to be determined. It appears doubtful that spirulina can compete with evening primrose in this respect. Unless and until further research reveals some good reason to spend money on spirulina, I recommend you skip it.

WHEAT GERM/ WHEAT-GERM OIL/ OCTACOSANOL

Many people consume wheat germ and the oil derived from it as sources of "natural" vitamin E and octacosanol. There is no persuasive evidence suggesting that vitamin E or any other substance derived from these sources is any more effective than vitamin E purchased in capsule form. The oil in these capsules, moreover, is far less likely to be rancid than that in the wheat germ.

Cureton has made an unconvincing argument based upon inadequate research (see T. K. Cureton, *The Physiological Effects of Wheat Germ Oil on Humans in Exercise*, Charles C. Thomas, Publisher, Springfield, Ill., 1972) that wheat-germ oil is superior to concentrated vitamin E supplements. The reason for this, he claims, is that the germ oil contains octacosanol, a 28 carbon alcohol. Manufacturers and promoters of wheat-germ oil now compete with one another on the basis of how much octacosanol their respective products contain. If they cared about the facts, rather than merely about luring the consumer, they'd save their breath. Even Cureton only *speculates* that octacosanol is the factor that supposedly improves the physical stamina and performance of those taking wheat-germ oil (rather than vitamin E in capsule form). The fact is there isn't a shred of scientific evidence anywhere that octacosanol plays any role in human biology and health.

It is interesting and instructive to note that those who write articles touting octacosanol frequently cite a particular scientific paper, clearly implying that this paper (*Proceedings of the New*

York Academy of Sciences, 33:(6)625, 1971) supports their claims; in fact, however, this paper is about the catalytic reagent dicobalt octacarbonyl, which has nothing to do with octacosanol!

One final note on this subject: It now appears that earlier discoveries showing a possible beneficial role of wheat-germ oil in the treatment of muscular dystrophy (*Journal of Neurology, Neurosurgery and Psychiatry*, 14:95, 1951) may have been due to an entirely different substance, such as selenium, which it now appears may play some role in this disorder, although this remains to be clearly demonstrated.

ten

PHARMACEUTICALS AND CHEMICALS

Though pharmaceutical drugs, both prescription and over-the-counter, are seldom thought of as "food supplements," a number of them are, in fact, increasingly being treated as such. Claims are being made that several drugs—and various chemical compounds not ordinarily found in food except when used as preservatives—have certain anti-aging effects. Anti-aging claims made for the following pharmaceuticals/chemicals are reviewed and analyzed in this chapter:

Aspirin
BHA and BHT
Deaner (DMAE)
DHEA
DMSO
L-dopa
Gerovital H3(GH3)
Hydergine

ASPIRIN

Aspirin an anti-aging agent? Very possibly, yes, at least in the sense that there is evidence that aspirin helps protect against some of the cardiovascular diseases that so often characterize aging. There have been numerous studies (see, for example, *Journal of the American Medical Association*, 243:661, 1980) suggesting, though not proving conclusively, that aspirin can help prevent the recurrence of heart attacks in those who have already suffered them and that it can reduce the death rate among heart-attack patients. The suggested mechanism (*Mayo Clinic Proceedings*, 56:102, 185, 265, 1981) by which aspirin exerts its protective effect is its ability to help block formation of blood clots. Such clots can obstruct the coronary arteries, reducing the flow of blood to the heart, causing chest pain (angina pectoris) and, often, heart attacks.

Recently, Lewis and co-workers presented the results of an aspirin study (*New England Journal of Medicine*, 309:396, 1983) that is far more conclusive than any of its predecessors. This study disclosed a definite protective effect in patients with severe angina pain. In this carefully controlled double-blind study, angina patients who received aspirin therapy (324 milligrams in buffered solution daily) had an incidence of acute heart attack and death 51 percent lower than similar angina patients who received placebos in the critical twelve-week period following hospitalization for unstable angina. Even a year later the aspirin group had a death rate 43 percent below that of the placebo group—despite the fact that aspirin was administered for only the first twelve weeks of that year. Nearly 1,300 patients from twelve different medical centers participated in the study, which has to be accounted a major one.

No significant side effects were noted in the study cited above. Aspirin was given, however, in a highly buffered water-soluble form. Gastrointestinal irritation and bleeding have often been reported in other studies in which higher doses of aspirin were given in tablet or capsule form. Even highly buffered aspirin in water-soluble form may, of course, prove troublesome if used for long periods of time. At present, only your doctor can determine whether you should take aspirin on a regular basis. Eventually, research may yield modified forms of aspirin that can safely be taken as preventive supplements. No such modified forms are available at the present time, though experimentation is under way. For now, use aspirin only according to the directions on the product label or as advised by a physician. This is an exciting area of research.

BHA AND BHT

Here's another case where some outrageous—and dangerous— claims have been made. BHA and BHT are both antioxidants that are commonly added in *minute* quantities to foods, especially oils and fats, as preservatives. (They are also used to preserve some plastics and rubber.) Recently, claims have been made that these chemicals control herpes infections, combat cancer and extend life-span. A couple of authors have suggested that gram and even higher daily doses of these substances are safe and effective against herpes. The best available scientific evidence does not support these claims; indeed, there is evidence indicating that the regular use of these chemicals in supplement form may pose very substantial health hazards.

Butylated hydroxyanisole (BHA) and butylated hydroxytoluene (BHT) have both exhibited some positive, as well as negative, qualities in small and preliminary studies. It is *possible* that one or both will eventually be shown to have value in the treatment of certain disorders under some circumstances. It is certain, however, that if that happens these substances will be treated as drugs and not as innocuous "food supplements." Here is one instance in which the nutritional "academic conservatives" can, with ample justification, accuse the nutritional "true believers" and some of the supplement manufacturers of extreme irresponsibility in promoting and selling poorly tested, highly potent nonnutritional substances, the perils of which are at least as well documented as the promises.

Both BHA and BHT are recognized antioxidants. Harman (*Age*, 3:100, 1980) has reported increased average life-span in long-lived strains of mice given BHT supplements. Increases as great as 30 percent were noted. Another mouse study (*Journal of Gerontology*, 28:415, 1973) indicated that large doses of vitamin E and BHT given in combination could inhibit the accumulation of "age pigments" in cells. At present there are

insufficient supporting data to assess the validity of these findings or to interpret their possible significance for humans.

As for cancer, the experimental data related to protective
claims are stronger with respect to BHA than to BHT. BHA has
been shown to inhibit chemically induced cancers in a number
of mouse and rat animal models. (See *Diet, Nutrition and Cancer*, National Academy Press, Washington, D.C., 1982, for a
review of these studies.) BHA, in several of these investigations,
has been shown to strongly increase the activity of an enzyme
called glutathione S-transferase, which has the ability to detoxify many chemical cancer-causing agents. Evidence that BHT
can also inhibit some cancers (*Journal of Investigative Dermatology*, 65:412, 1975; *Age*, 1:162, 1978) is in far shorter supply.

There is, in fact, a growing body of evidence suggesting that
BHT can *promote* the growth of some cancers. Witschi and
colleagues (*Toxicology*, 21:37, 1981), working with mice, showed
that BHT promotes the growth of lung cancers caused by three
chemical carcinogens. Other work by Witschi alone (*Toxicology*, 21:95, 1981) and in collaboration with others (*Journal of the
National Cancer Institute*, 58:301, 1977) has shown that the
incidence of lung tumors increases even when BHT is not given
to test animals until as late as five months after the cancer-
initiating chemical is injected. BHT, therefore, does not appear
to be a primary cause of these cancers but, rather, encourages
and boosts the growth of cancer once it gets started. Dr. Alvin
Malkinson of the University of Colorado School of Pharmacy
advised the FDA in 1983 that he has confirmed tumor-promot-
ing effects of BHT in various strains of mice. A recent report by
Maeura et al. (*American Association of Cancer Research Abstracts*, 1983, p. 87) showed that although BHT inhibited liver
cancer in rats exposed to a carcinogenic agent, it promoted
bladder cancer.

Claims have been made that BHT can protect against herpes
and other viruses. The relevant scientific data (*Science*, 188:64,
1975; *Journal of Infectious Diseases*, 138:91, 1978) relate to in
vitro (test tube) inactivation by BHT of various lipid-containing
viruses, including herpes simplex and cytomegalovirus. But
what applies in vitro often does not apply in vivo (in the living
body), and at present there is no proof that BHT can inactivate
any virus in humans. The claim that BHT can in very large
doses prevent outbreaks of herpes is purely anecdotal. And even

these positive anecdotes are countered by negative ones. I personally know people who have taken large doses of BHT daily in hope of warding off herpes attacks or of shortening the duration and intensity of those attacks once they developed; they report that BHT was ineffective in every respect. There is absolutely no scientific justification for using BHT to try to prevent or treat herpes; and to do so, as outlined above, may entail some serious risk.

Apart from the cancer risks, the use of BHT poses some other perils. Allergic reactions, though admittedly isolated ones, have been reported (*British Journal of Dermatology*, 94:233, 1976) to even the small quantities of BHT that have been added to some foods as preservatives. In a review of earlier work by himself and Denz, Llaurado reports (*Western Journal of Medicine*, 139:229, 1983) on "dramatic deleterious effects" of *both* BHA and BHT in controlled experimental studies in which rabbits received 1 gram of BHA or BHT daily, with resulting muscular weakness, damage to kidneys and adrenal glands, and death. "Daily doses of 1 gram given to rabbits were lethal in about two weeks," Llaurado notes. "In terms of concentration of drug per kg of animal mass, the . . . dose of 2 grams a day [that some BHT enthusiasts have recommended as a genital-herpes preventative] is simply *one order of magnitude* below the lethal dose. Obviously, smaller doses, if not lethal, must produce pathological effects."

Clearly, some researchers are convinced that BHT and BHA are very dangerous substances. We still do not have enough information to make *absolutely conclusive* judgments about this. But until we do—and in view of BHT's widely demonstrated cancer-promoting properties—the prudent consumer will keep a healthy distance from either of these potent chemicals when they are offered as food supplements. The prudent consumer would also do well to keep a healthy distance from those individuals who promote these potentially dangerous substances as food supplements, antiherpes treatment and so on.

DEANER (DMAE)

"Deaner" and "Deanol" are the registered names of prescription drugs that contain dimethylaminoethanol (DMAE), thought by some to be a precursor of acetylcholine (see discussion of choline elsewhere in this book). Like choline, DMAE has been used to treat various disorders of the nervous system. It appears to have a beneficial role in the treatment of tardive dyskinesia and Huntington's chorea (*Pharmacology, Biochemistry and Behavior*, 15:285, 1981). There is no support, however, for recent claims that DMAE is a potent life extender that might benefit the general population. The life-spans of some animals were reported (*Experimental Gerontology*, 8:177, 1973) to have been extended through DMAE supplementation, but a more recent study not only failed to confirm this but *found the opposite to be true*. Deanol-treated animals actually had *shorter* life-spans than control animals that did not receive this substance. Some have noted the relationship of DMAE to Gerovital H3 (see analysis later in this chapter), one of the breakdown products of which is diethylaminoethanol (DEAE), a close chemical relative. If DMAE has an efficacy at all it appears likely that this is due to its role as a choline precursor in the liver. (See *Brain Acetylcholine and Neuropsychiatric Disease*, Plenum Press, New York, 1979, p. 483.) The choline synthesized in the liver from DMAE can go to the brain via the blood and may play a role in the regulation of acetylcholine there. No such role can be conceived of for DEAE.

Deaner is a prescription drug with very limited application. It certainly should not be used as a dietary supplement, as some "life extension" enthusiasts have suggested. As noted above, in the best animal study of this substance to date, DMAE actually shortened, rather than lengthened, life-span!

DHEA

It wasn't long ago that the hormone dehydroepiandrosterone (DHEA) was strictly the stuff of experimental medicine. Now, suddenly, it is available in vitamin stores and advertised in multicolor brochures featuring bikini-clad beauties who, we are apparently to believe, came by their svelte shapes and satisfied smiles via regular ingestion of a DHEA product that, the brochures declare, is compounded from "bovine tissue and specially imported Mexican yams." According to the claims, regular ingestion of DHEA supplements will inhibit weight gain and, it is implied, extend life-span and reduce the incidence of various cancers.

All of these claims are extrapolated from limited but interesting experimental animal data. That animal research was stimulated by the observation of Bulbrook (*Lancet*, 2:395, 1971) that some women with breast cancer had lower than normal levels of two substances that are derived mainly from DHEA, which is a steroid hormone produced in relatively large quantities by the adrenal glands of mammals, including man. This led Schwartz and co-workers (*Cancer Research*, 35:2482, 1975, 39:1129, 1979; *Nutrition and Cancer*, 3:46, 1981) to conduct a number of animal experiments which suggested that DHEA might be protective against some cancers. Mice that normally develop breast tumors were slower to develop them when treated with DHEA. But note that the tumors did, in fact, still develop. Subsequent, unconfirmed work by Schwartz et al. indicates that DHEA may also have some protective effect against lung and colon cancers. There are, as yet, no convincing data that DHEA can significantly extend life-span in experimental animals, but Schwartz and others have reported that DHEA-treated animals that are obese to begin with often lose weight without reducing food intake.

Suggested mechanisms for DHEA's possible anticancer, antiobesity effects include its hypothesized ability to inhibit an enzyme that is involved in the production of fat and of substances that may promote chemical carcinogenesis. Much is made in the health-food literature of the fact that blood levels of DHEA decline with age in humans. Thus, it is argued, we need to "replace" what is lost with supplements. Such arguments are, at best, premature.

First, there is still no evidence that the animal data (which, in any event, have yet to be widely and thoroughly confirmed) will have any bearing on human health. Second, there is no guarantee at this point that long-term DHEA supplementation will be safe. DHEA is a precursor to the sex hormones, e.g., testosterone, and could increase the risk of prostate cancer. No one knows yet what the long-term effects might be. Third, the DHEA products being sold are unlikely to have any positive effects; most of this oral DHEA will be broken down in the liver and will never reach the cells that it is supposed to rejuvenate. The doses used in the animal work were enormous compared with anything any reasonably sane human consumer would want to risk at a time when our knowledge of this substance is imperfect, to say the least. Hold off on this one until more—and better—information is available.

DMSO

"DMSO may be a passé wonder drug, but it still gathers the faithful." So said *Medical World News* (Oct. 11, 1982, p. 30). It's still difficult to pass health-food outlets or even many hardware and army-surplus stores without seeing a sign that circumspectly declares: "DMSO." Meaning: DMSO sold *here*. Dimethyl sulfoxide (DMSO) has been used since the 1940s as an industrial solvent. Jacob and co-workers introduced it into therapeutic practice in the 1960s (*American Journal of Surgery*, 114:414, 1967), and it has since then been used by tens of thousands of individuals as a treatment, applied topically, for strains, sprains, bruises and arthritis.

After once banning research on DMSO out of fear that the chemical might cause serious eye damage, the FDA later allowed investigations to continue and, in 1978, approved the use of DMSO to treat the symptoms of interstitial cystitis (fibrosis of the bladder wall, occurring primarily in women over forty). DMSO is being studied—but has not been approved—for use in a number of skin, nerve and autoimmune diseases. It is also being studied to see what effect it might have on some forms of cancer. The FDA is monitoring thirty or more DMSO studies. In some of these, the substance is being administered intravenously to test i.s effects on brain-injured patients, victims of spinal-cord injury and cerebral stroke. Some studies have turned up negative findings but, at the same time, have not reported serious side effects, either to eyes or kidneys, following long-term, *low-dose* DMSO treatment. There is some preliminary evidence (see review by Martin, *Critical Care Quarterly*, Mar. 1983, p. 72) that intravenous DMSO may have some usefulness in the treatment of brain-injured individuals; but, as the author of this review notes, the use of DMSO for this purpose —as for most others—remains speculative pending well-controlled studies of the sort that have largely been lacking to date.

Weaver and colleagues (reported upon in Oregon Health Sciences University's *Second Annual Research Convocation Exhibit Synopses*, No. 20, Portland, Nov. 1983) found that a 3 percent concentration of DMSO in the drinking water of a strain of mice that spontaneously develop a serious disease syndrome had significant beneficial effects. The mice studied have a gene that gives rise to tumors of the lymph nodes and autoimmune diseases resembling systemic lupus and rheumatoid arthritis. Some 90 percent of those mice given DMSO in their drinking water, commencing at ten weeks of age, were still alive at forty weeks, according to the report of these researchers, while only 50 percent of the control mice, which did not get DMSO in their water, were alive at twenty weeks. There were far fewer tumors among the forty-week-old survivors than among the twenty-week-old controls. Another set of mice—all older and already in advanced stages of disease when started on DMSO-laced drinking water at seven months of age—exhibited significant tumor-mass regression after the DMSO was introduced. Levels of autoantibodies against DNA (of the sort implicated in some autoimmune syndromes) were diminished in DMSO-treated mice. These intriguing findings need follow-up.

DMSO may have antioxidant properties, but this has not yet been established. The proposed modes of action of DMSO are almost as numerous as its claimed benefits; none of these modes has been widely accepted. This, however, has not stopped nearly a dozen states from permitting doctors to prescribe DMSO for various ailments. Certainly no one should use DMSO without a doctor's prescription and then only after asking to see the evidence that the substance is effective in the ailment in question. The DMSO that is being sold in many storefronts and on the street should be avoided; it is almost never of the relatively pure grade used in clinical trials. Contaminants pose a real risk.

L-DOPA

Recent suggestions that even generally healthy people might benefit from regular use of the amino acid L-dopa, a prescription drug, are unfounded and very likely dangerous. "Life-extension" enthusiasts like to cite the study of Cotzias and co-workers (*Proceedings of the National Academy of Sciences*, 71:2469, 1974) as evidence that L-dopa is a miraculous rejuvenator. Cotzias did, in fact, report that the life-spans of some mice were substantially extended after gradual adaptation to large doses of L-dopa. This is an interesting study—and one that should be followed up—but it is not a study that supports the argument that *humans* should start taking this powerful substance on a routine basis; neither does it support the claim that L-dopa is a life extender in humans or even, in the absence of well-controlled confirmation, in mice. It is well to note too that in the Cotzias study a number of mice given sudden, large doses of L-dopa died.

L-dopa is used, with some success, in the treatment of Parkinson's disease, a condition characterized by partial loss of motor control with resulting tremor. The biochemical disorders implicated in this disease are sometimes favorably modified by the administration of L-dopa, which promotes the production of dopamine, a brain neurotransmitter often found to be in short supply in Parkinsonism. Findings (*American Journal of Psychiatry*, 135:1552, 1978) that sexual function is sometimes enhanced in male victims of Parkinson's via L-dopa treatment suggest, in addition, an effect on the hormonal processes involved in this function. Some slight, inconclusive evidence has been found (*British Medical Journal*, Mar. 4, 1978, p. 550) that L-dopa might have a favorable effect on senile dementia in some patients.

Overall, the evidence that L-dopa can be of benefit outside of Parkinson's disease is unconvincing. Contradictory effects are continually being reported with this drug. Adverse effects match positive ones. Depression and nausea are commonly reported side effects of L-dopa. There are also more serious side effects. This is not a drug to be taken lightly.

GEROVITAL H3 (GH3)

Gerovital H3 (GH3) is a procaine preparation first developed and promoted as an anti-aging agent by Dr. Ana Aslan, director of the Institute of Geriatrics in Bucharest, Rumania. According to the Rumanian National Tourist Office, the Aslan clinic has treated "world-renowned actors, actresses, writers and statesmen," who have had conferred upon them, in the process, "the secret of eternal vigor and youth." Well, the first part of that, at least, is true. Numerous prominent individuals still make annual and semiannual pilgrimages to Rumania in search of the fountain of youth—and to be certain that they get the "original," the "authentic" Aslan formula. Others settle for procaine products packaged in Mexico or produced in Nevada, one of the few U.S. locations where it can be legally dispensed.

As for the "eternal vigor and youth," don't get your hopes up. Claims that GH3 and its imitators can extend life-span, rejuvenate skin and hair, halt and even reverse senility, increase sexual potency, overcome arthritis, protect against cardiovascular disease and nervous disorders have, without exception, proved false. Studies claiming to demonstrate these effects are few in number and inadequate in design; most are uncontrolled or poorly controlled. (See review of the literature by Ostfeld et al., *Journal of the American Geriatric Society*, 25:1, 1977; also a more recent review by Thomas, *Medical Journal of Australia*, June 11, 1983, p. 543.) When adequately controlled studies *have* been conducted, they have failed to support the claims made for this substance (*Medical Letter*, Jan. 12, 1979, p. 4).

GH3 is a 2 percent procaine hydrochloride solution to which minute amounts of the following have been added as "stabilizers" or "buffers": benzoic acid, potassium metabisulfite and disodium phosphate. The procaine (which is the same as the novocaine anesthetic that you get when you go to the dentist) is supposed to be the active ingredient. However, as Thomas (cited above) notes, procaine is rapidly hydrolyzed (decomposed) once it enters the bloodstream, even after buffering or stabilizing agents are added, and there is no evidence—or even any good reason to suspect—that these additives can sustain the activity of procaine long enough to produce the claimed benefits. Of course, some have theorized that the breakdown products—primarily para-aminobenzoic acid (PABA) and diethylaminoethanol (DEAE)—are the active ingredients. The problem with this argument is that neither of these substances has been shown to possess the miraculous powers claimed for GH3 (see discussions elsewhere in this book of PABA and DMAE, which is chemically related to DEAE). Moreover, the amounts of these substances that result from the breakdown of GH3 are extremely small.

Claims, taken seriously for a time by many researchers, that GH3 is an effective antidepressant, especially in the aged, have failed to be confirmed. It was claimed that procaine could inhibit the formation of a brain chemical—monoamine oxidase (MAO)—that has been associated with depression. Jarvik and co-workers (in S. Gershon and A. Raksin, eds., *Aging*, Vol. 2, Raven Press, New York, 1975) found that GH3 was neither more nor less effective than placebo in counteracting depression.

There is no evidence that GH3 has any effect on aging. Adverse side effects infrequently occur and include allergic reactions, abrupt drop in blood pressure, respiratory difficulty and convulsions. Some of these reactions may be due to contaminants in some of the products, the costs of which, incidentally, are often very substantial. GH3 is not recommended under any circumstances.

HYDERGINE

Sandoz has developed a drug containing a mixture of dihydrogenated ergot alkaloids that it calls Hydergine. Though still little known in the United States, Hydergine is one of the most prescribed drugs worldwide. Claims for it are broad but focus primarily on its effects on the brain and nervous system. Hydergine is said to retard aging of the brain, improve memory, counteract senility and, generally, keep the gray matter humming optimally. Possible modes of action of Hydergine have been reviewed by Yesavage and group (*Journal of the American Geriatrics Society*, 27:80, 1979). Hydergine affects enzyme systems that are involved in the electrochemistry of nerve signals. There is evidence that Hydergine increases the level of nerve-signal message transmission, especially at dopamine and serotonin receptor sites in the brain. Completely unsubstantiated claims have been made that Hydergine can increase intelligence in normal people. There's even a claim it can revive the "recently dead." More down-to-earth claims have some validity.

Lazzari and co-workers (*Aging*, 23:347, 1983) cite numerous controlled clinical double-blind trials of Hydergine showing benefit in cases of "chronic senile cerebral insufficiency" (CSCI), a form of diminished mental capacity characterized by confusion, loss of short-term memory, disorientation, depression, etc., and caused by various aging processes, including narrowing of the blood vessels to the brain. In this interim report on their own long-term double-blind Hydergine study, by far the best-designed to date, Lazzari et al. confirm and expand the positive findings related to the use of this drug in the treatment of CSCI.

More than 400 patients are being treated at more than forty centers in Italy. Results to date are highly encouraging. Patients receiving 1.5-milligram tablets of Hydergine twice daily have consistently performed substantially better on a number of subjective and objective tests related to mood, memory and cognition than have control patients receiving placebos. The conclusion of Lazzari and co-workers is: "Hydergine has an important place among the drugs of which we are speaking and it is widely used, but its action is not yet fully accepted or believed. The results after six months of therapy with Hydergine, in this double-blind, placebo-controlled clinical trial, open a new horizon and convince us."

These researchers termed the results obtained "remarkable" but added that in most cases three months of Hydergine therapy are required before significant improvement begins to be evident. They caution, as well, that the long-term effects of Hydergine remain to be elucidated. There is always the possibility that the observed benefits will eventually fade even with continued administration of the drug—or that some serious adverse side effect, so far absent, will manifest itself.

Hydergine is, at this point, a very promising substance that may eventually be shown to have a protective role against dementia. There is not enough good information available, as yet, however, to justify recommending use of this drug as a preventive supplement, as some have done. It is far too early to say what the long-term effects, either positive or negative, of this substance may be. The underground traffic in Hydergine is unfortunate and may seriously impede legitimate research. This is a prescription drug that should be used only in accordance with its approved use.

In the United States Hydergine is prescribed at doses no higher than 1 milligram three times daily. Physicians in the U.S. are presently restricted to this limit for the treatment of Alzheimer's-like dementia, which is the most common form of pre-senile dementia. There is some indication that if this drug is started in the early stages of this disorder, but not in the advanced stages, some improvement in memory may result.

PART THREE

RECOM-
MENDA-
TIONS/
CONSUMER
INFORMA-
TION

*Recommended
Regimens and
Guidelines*

eleven

RECOMMENDED REGIMENS FOR DIFFERENT LIFE SITUATIONS

The following regimens are *suggestions* for people in different categories. Use these regimens as general information to help guide you in the right direction. Some information on specific products, which may help further serve as models of what to look for, is contained in the next chapter of this book.

Note that these regimens are for vitamins, minerals and trace elements. For recommendations on other food supplements, miscellaneous chemicals and various pharmaceuticals for which anti-aging claims have been made, many of which may relate to specific life situations, see analyses of individual substances in Part Two of this book.

Note that at the end of this chapter there is a section called Drug/Vitamin/Mineral Interactions. *All supplement users should read this section in order to avoid mixtures of drugs/ supplements that are potentially dangerous or that negate the effects of either the drugs or the nutrients.*

Basic Regimen for Men

Overview

It is still believed by many that generally healthy individuals do not require vitamin and mineral supplementation so long as they eat adequate amounts of a well-balanced diet. I agree that it is highly unlikely that the signs and symptoms of *gross* vitamin- and mineral-deficiency states will occur in such individuals. Nonetheless, I believe it to be prudent for even "healthy" people to take a daily vitamin and mineral supplement for maximum nutritional insurance. The reasons for this are made evident in preceding chapters.

We really do not yet know the optimal vitamin and mineral requirements for maximum health and longevity. Accumulating evidence is showing us that the very foods we eat in our "well-balanced" diet may contain substances that produce such degenerative diseases as cancer. Interestingly, many of these substances produce their effects by the generation of toxic forms of oxygen. Several of the vitamins and minerals participate in the *detoxification* of these dangerous entities. These vitamin and mineral antioxidants may also be protective against other forms of degenerative diseases, such as cardiovascular diseases and osteoarthritis. A vitamin and mineral "insurance" supplement is recommended for healthy individuals as a key element in the prevention of many of these degenerative diseases.

The following Basic Regimen is the one I recommend for most healthy men. The contents and amounts, as well as the recommended form, are derived from the studies that are analyzed in this book. Admittedly, these recommended amounts are, at best, approximations of what appears optimal at this time; it is expected that in the future further research of this vital matter will yield more definitive data. The reader should review all the material in preceding chapters related to each nutrient before following this or any of the suggested regimens. Special attention should be paid to any noted "precautions."

The Basic Regimen for Men omits iron since even a marginal iron deficiency in men who eat more than 2,000 calories per day is suggestive of a pathological process that requires medical investigation.

Note that none of the vitamins or minerals are present in megadose amounts, that is, in amounts greater than ten times the U.S. RDA. I believe that a *well-balanced* vitamin/mineral supplement obviates the need for megadose supplementation. For example, selenium and zinc, present in the right balance and amounts, adequately spare the antioxidant activity of vitamin E, making intake of amounts of vitamin E much greater than 200 IU daily unnecessary and unjustified. A well-balanced supplement is a highly *efficient* supplement, and that is what I have strived for here and in all of these regimens.

I recommend that the daily supplement be taken in divided doses. Splitting it into three doses, one with each meal, is ideal. Some of the antioxidant protection afforded by this supplement may take place before the supplement is absorbed into the bloodstream. Many of the foods we eat contain substances that cause free-radical damage. Antioxidant protection with each meal could help prevent this damage in the stomach and intestines.

The Regimen

This is the Basic Regimen for Men—a daily vitamin and mineral supplement for adequate nutritional insurance. (Pay attention to milligrams (mg) and micrograms (mcg). There's a *big* difference.)

Basic Regimen for Women (Premenopausal Women Not on the Pill)

Overview

The micronutritional regimen I recommend for this group is similar to the Basic Regimen for Men, with the exception of iron. Since premenopausal women have a monthly blood loss as well as a lower iron reserve than men, it is prudent for them to take an insurance supplement of iron, especially if they have

TABLE 2

VITAMINS	RECOMMENDED FORM	AMOUNT	% U.S. RDA
Vitamin A	beta-carotene	20,000 IU	400
Vitamin B$_1$	thiamine	10 mg	667
Vitamin B$_2$	riboflavin	10 mg	588
Niacinamide	niacinamide	100 mg	500
Pantothenic Acid	calcium pantothenate	50 mg	500
Vitamin B$_6$	pyridoxine	10 mg	500
Vitamin B$_{12}$	cyanoco- balamin	6 mcg	100
Biotin	biotin	100 mcg	33
Folic Acid	folic acid	400 mcg	100
Vitamin C	ascorbic acid	500 mg	833
Vitamin E	d-alpha toco- pheryl acetate	200 IU	667
Vitamin D$_3$	cholecalciferol	400 IU	100

MINERALS			
Calcium	carbonate	1,000 mg	100
Copper	gluconate	2 mg	100
Chromium	organic form/ chromium yeast	100 mcg	*
Magnesium	gluconate preferred/ oxide acceptable	400 mg	100
Manganese	gluconate	5 mg	*
Molybdenum	sodium molybdate	50 mcg	*
Selenium	organic form/ selenium yeast	200 mcg	*
Zinc	gluconate	15 mg	100
Iodine	potassium iodide	150 mcg	100

* U.S. RDA not determined but essentially established.

heavier than normal menstrual flow or they are fitted with IUDs, which may predispose to additional blood loss.

Ideally, iron should be taken by itself between meals for maximum absorption. Iron in the form of ferrous sulfate is the best form (cheapest and most readily absorbed). Some, however, may find ferrous sulfate irritating to the gastrointestinal tract and may thus prefer ferrous fumarate, which is entirely acceptable. Those women who take their iron in a multivitamin/multimineral preparation should be aware that calcium decreases the bioavailability of iron. Ascorbic acid, on the other hand, increases it.

The Regimen

Same as the Basic Regimen for Men except:

Add iron, in the form of sulfate or fumarate, in the amount of 18 mg daily, which is 100% of the U.S. RDA.

Regimen for Women Using Oral Contraceptives

Overview

There is evidence that women who use oral contraceptives have decreased vitamin B_6 (pyridoxine) and folic acid. The mood changes, typically depression, that many women who use oral contraceptives experience have been attributed to decreased synthesis of the neurotransmitter serotonin. This decreased synthesis may be a consequence of decreased vitamin B_6 status.

The regimen I recommend here is the same as the Basic Regimen for Women (the premenopausal regimen) except that in addition to the iron which is added in that regimen, I also recommend doubling the daily B_6 intake to 20 milligrams to insure maintenance of a normal vitamin B_6 status.

The Regimen

Same as Basic Regimen for Women except:

Add an additional 10 mg of vitamin B_6 daily, bringing the total to 20 mg of B_6 daily.

Regimen for Pregnant Women

Overview

Pregnant women have additional requirements for most of the micronutrients, particularly folic acid and iron. In the case of iron, it is highly unlikely that pregnant women can obtain iron from the foods they eat in sufficient quantities to prevent iron deficiency. It is thus recommended that pregnant women take 60 milligrams of supplementary iron daily. Some pregnant women may require more than this. Every pregnant woman should be carefully evaluated by her obstetrician to determine the amount of iron needed to prevent deficiency.

The best form of iron is ferrous sulfate, although ferrous fumarate is also acceptable and may be better tolerated by many women. Iron is best absorbed on an empty stomach and, ideally, should be taken *about one hour before a meal*. Many women, however, suffer gastric irritation when they take iron on an empty stomach. If switching to the fumarate form doesn't alleviate this irritation, then take your iron with meals.

Iron contained in a multivitamin/multimineral preparation that includes calcium may lead to iron's decreased absorption.

Supplementary folic acid is recommended at a daily dose of 800 to 1,000 micrograms.

Vitamins A and E are used at lower doses here than in the Basic Regimen for Women. The probability of any adverse effects from these vitamins on the fetus is very low even at the higher doses, but as a precaution the doses are lowered here. This regimen should be used only after discussion with your obstetrician.

The Regimen

Same as the Basic Regimen for Women except:

1) Take 10,000 IU of Vitamin A (in the form of beta-carotene only) daily. This is *half* of the amount recommended in the Basic Regimen for Women. The reason for the reduction is explained above.

2) Reduce niacinamide intake from 100 mg to 50 mg.
3) Take 800 to 1,000 mcg of folic acid daily instead of the 400 mcg recommended in the Basic Regimen for Women.
4) Reduce, for reasons explained above, your daily supplemental intake of Vitamin E to 60 IU—instead of the 200 IU recommended in the Basic Regimen for Women.
5) Put your total iron intake at 60 mg daily, unless otherwise advised by your physician. Some women may need more than this in supplemental form.
6) Increase your calcium intake to 1,300 mg daily, instead of the 1,000 recommended in the Basic Regimen for Women. (Consult the Basic Regimen for proper form of each nutrient.)
7) Put your total daily supplemental magnesium intake at 450 mg.

Regimen for Postmenopausal Women

Overview

Osteoporosis, a bone disease characterized by decreased bone density, increased brittleness of bone and loss of bone calcium, is not uncommon in postmenopausal women. There is evidence that supplementary calcium (1.5 grams daily) may help in the prevention of this disease (see analysis of calcium in Part Two).

The regimen I recommend for postmenopausal women includes 1.5 grams of calcium (as carbonate). Other components, the same as in the Basic Regimen for Men, afford the antioxidant protection needed by this group. Iron supplementation is *not* recommended for this group. Iron deficiency in postmenopausal women should be investigated by a physician as it may represent a pathological process.

Postmenopausal women with hypercalcemia (high concentrations of calcium in the blood) should avoid calcium supplementation. Postmenopausal women with kidney failure should not take magnesium supplementation. Postmenopausal women taking estrogens need take only 1 gram of calcium daily.

The Regimen

Same as the Basic Regimen for Women except:

1) Increase calcium, in the form of calcium carbonate, to a total of 1,500 mg daily. See precautions above.
2) Do not take iron supplementation unless your physician approves.

Regimen for People on Weight-Loss Diets

Overview

As the numbers of calories are reduced in the diet so are the amounts of vitamins and minerals. Weight-loss diets that restrict calories have become popular as the prevalence of obesity in developed countries has increased. Recently, very-low-calorie diets, low in carbohydrates and fat and high in protein, have become very popular. These are the "protein-sparing," modi-fied-fast (liquid protein) diets. All low-calorie and in particular the very-low-calorie diets place those using them at increased risk of vitamin and mineral deficiencies.

In fact, mineral deficiencies have been implicated in deaths resulting from the prolonged use of some of these very-low-calorie diets (diets with fewer than 500 calories per day) in peo-ple *not* supplementing these diets with vitamins and minerals. It was first thought that inadequate potassium was responsible for the cardiac arrhythmias (abnormal heart rhythm) believed to be the cause of death in individuals on these diets. It is now thought that inadequate intake of other minerals, as well as of potassium, played a role in these deaths.

Apart from all that, the mere process of burning fat, which occurs at accelerated rates during weight reduction, can gener-ate significant free-radical activity, which, as discussed earlier, can cause a lot of damage to tissue. Since many of the vitamins and minerals protect against such damage, those who restrict calories, i.e., go on weight-loss diets, are at increased risk of free-radical-mediated tissue damage and accelerated aging.

I recommend that all individuals using very-low-calorie weight-loss diets do so *only under the close supervision of a physician who is an expert in the use of these diets.* Continuous monitoring should be carried out to ensure that no vitamin or mineral deficiencies occur.

The regimen recommended here, however, is designed for people on weight-loss diets of all types. Vitamin K_1 (phylloquinone) is added because of reports that those on very-low-calorie diets may have increased bleeding tendencies due to deficiency in this particular vitamin. Iron is included since low-calorie diets tend to be deficient in this mineral. Biotin is increased because some of the weight-loss diets are high in egg-white protein, which can cause biotin deficiency, sometimes manifested by hair loss. Potassium is included since very-low-calorie diets commonly lead to potassium-deficiency states. People on those very-low-calorie diets should have their serum potassium checked by their physicians to ensure that they receive appropriate potassium replacement.

The Regimen

Same as the Basic Regimen for Men except:

1) Increase biotin to a total of 300 mcg per day.
2) Add 100 mcg of vitamin K_1 (phylloquinone).
3) Add iron (in the form of sulfate or fumarate) for a total of 18 mg daily.
4) Add the mineral potassium, in the form of potassium chloride, for a total of 860 mg daily. *Do not exceed this amount except on advice of your physician.*

Regimen for Smokers (And Nonsmokers Exposed to Cigarette Smoke)

Overview

There is evidence that many of the toxic elements in cigarette smoke are oxidants—generators of toxic oxygen forms that can cause molecular, cellular and tissue damage. Cigarette smoke contains high amounts of nitrogen oxides, which are themselves free radicals. Nitrogen oxides can react with polyunsaturated fatty acids, which are found in cellular membranes; this reaction commonly leads to premature death. Vitamin E, in particular, protects against these reactions.

The cancer-causing potential of cigarette smoking is well established. Lung cancer, associated with smoking, accounts for more cancer deaths than any other form of malignancy. Again, it is the free-radical activity that is believed to be the basic carcinogenic factor in smoking. Nonsmokers can also be significantly affected by the noxious agents in cigarette smoke. One recent study (see the April 1984 issue of *Western Journal of Medicine*) found that the wives of husbands who smoke, for example, died of cancer at twice the rate of wives whose husbands don't smoke. People who work in offices and other workplaces where smoking is permitted are also at increased risk.

Smokers and nonsmokers regularly exposed to cigarette smoke could certainly benefit from increased antioxidant protection. (Many of the risks of smoking, however, will still persist.) Such protection is afforded by substances such as vitamin A (beta-carotene), vitamin E, ascorbic acid (vitamin C), zinc, copper, selenium and magnesium. The following regimen takes these increased requirements into account; it also takes into account the fact that the cadmium present in cigarette *paper* antagonizes zinc, thus requiring an increase in that mineral and adjustment in copper intake.

The Regimen

Same as the Basic Regimens for Men and Women except:

1) Increase ascorbic acid (vitamin C) intake to a total of 1,000 mg daily (1 gram).
2) Increase vitamin E intake to a total of 400 IU daily.
3) Increase copper intake to a total of 3 mg daily.
4) Increase zinc intake to a total of 30 mg daily.

Regimen for Runners and Other Athletes

Overview

Energy is defined as the ability to do work. Runners, athletes and all persons performing exercise necessarily are doing more physical work than those who live more sedentary lives. The energy that is required for these activities is derived from the burning of the foodstuffs, carbohydrates, fats and proteins, to produce the carrier of biological energy, the molecule known as adenosine triphosphate, or ATP. ATP is mainly produced by the process known as oxidative phosphorylation. We now know that during this process a certain amount of free-radical toxic oxygen forms are produced and that this amount probably increases the more this process is used. We may thus expect that those engaged in regular exercise will produce increased amounts of free-radical activity.

The regimen that follows focuses on vitamins, minerals and, especially, the antioxidants that can put out some of the free-radical fires. Potassium is added because this mineral is lost in perspiration.

The Regimen

The Basic Regimens for Men and Women should prove adequate except:

Add 860 mg of potassium chloride daily.

And those interested in substances for which claims have been made with respect to increased stamina, muscle building, etc. should review Part Two again, looking, for example, at analyses of such substances as arginine, ornithine, carnitine, ginseng, pangamic acid, garlic, bee pollen, coenzyme Q, glandulars, octacosanol, DHEA, etc.

Regimen for Alcohol Drinkers

Overview

The active ingredient in alcoholic beverages is the substance ethanol. The alcohols are a family of organic substances, but the word "alcohol" is usually applied to the most famous member of this family—ethanol. Ethanol is capable of affecting physiological processes in many and complicated ways. Some of the breakdown products of ethanol metabolism in the body can produce free radicals; it is believed that this is the mechanism that underlies many of the toxic effects of alcohol.

The occasional, light consumer of alcohol should be able to get sufficient micronutritional "insurance" protection by using the Basic Regimens outlined above. Chronic alcohol users, however, commonly suffer from both micro- and macronutritional deficiencies. They are often characterized by insufficient/unbalanced intake of nutrients. The toxic effects of alcohol, moreover, reduce the ability to absorb and properly utilize nutrients.

Vitamins and minerals that are known to be depleted in chronic alcoholics include vitamins A, B_1, B_2, B_6, B_{12}, niacin, folic acid, vitamin C (ascorbic acid), vitamin D, magnesium, calcium, zinc and iron. Vitamin/mineral supplementation in alcoholics should include these substances as well as afford antioxidant protection, since much of the toxic damage of ethanol appears to be mediated by free radicals. Protection against free-radical damage is provided, to some extent, by supplemental vitamins A, C and E and by the minerals manganese, copper, selenium, zinc and magnesium.

The following regimen should give micronutritional protection for chronic consumers of alcohol. It is to be noted that vitamin B_1 (thiamine) is recommended at 100 milligrams daily and folic acid at from 800 to 1,000 micrograms daily to prevent deficiencies in these B vitamins. This regimen by itself will not protect against malnutrition in alcoholics. (That will require adequate and balanced intake of calories from protein, fats and carbohydrates.) The best way for the alcoholic to protect himself against malnutrition is, of course, to stop consuming alcohol. Nor should the alcoholic believe that by taking this regimen he will mitigate most of the damages of alcoholism. The regimen may help, but continued alcoholism is still likely to prove highly detrimental. And it should be remembered that those who both smoke and drink are at even greater risk of premature death from cancer, heart disease, etc.

The Regimen

The same as the Basic Regimens for Men and Women except:

1) Increase daily intake of vitamin B_1 (thiamine) to a total of 100 mg.
2) Increase daily intake of folic acid to a total of 800 to 1,000 mcg.
3) Increase daily intake of ascorbic acid (vitamin C) to a total of 1,000 mg (1 gram).
4) Increase daily intake of vitamin E to a total of 400 IU.
5) Increase daily copper intake to a total of 3 mg.
6) Increase daily intake of zinc to a total of 30 mg.

Consult Part Two for other substances that may offer protection against the toxic effects of alcohol. See, for example, analyses of wheatgrass, barley grass and other green plants.

Regimen for Hospitalized Patients (Surgical and Medical)

Overview

During the past ten years, several studies have shown that a surprisingly high percentage of hospitalized patients suffer from malnutrition (protein-calorie deficiencies as well as vitamin deficiencies), and this appears to worsen the longer these patients remain in the hospital. This is very detrimental to the patient's progress since optimal nutrition should be basic in the treatment of any surgical or medical problem. Fortunately, awareness of this situation is growing, so that the patient's nutritional status is being given more and better attention in many hospitals than ever before. This is particularly true of diet as a whole, that is with respect to the protein, carbohydrate, fat content of the diet, as well as to total calories in the diet. Only recently has attention been given to micronutrient content of diet—vitamins, minerals.

The following regimen is recommended for hospitalized patients who don't drink or smoke. (The latter should see applicable regimens.) You should consult with your physician, if possible, about vitamin/mineral supplementation prior to entering the hospital. Depending upon the reason for hospitalization, your doctor may want to make modifications in this regimen, either increasing or decreasing certain constituents. Magnesium, for example, should be withheld from patients with renal (kidney) failure. Calcium should be withheld from patients with hypercalcemia. The recommended regimen can be given either in tablet or powder form (mixed in milk, juices), convenient for those patients who have trouble swallowing pills. There are a number of vitamins, minerals and other nutritional substances that may help speed healing of injuries, surgical wounds and so on. Zinc has been found to be useful in patients who tend to heal slowly, especially when given in relatively high doses (about 150 milligrams daily). These higher doses, however, should be taken only under a doctor's supervision.

The Regimen

Same as the Basic Regimens for Men and Women except:

1) Increase total daily copper intake to 3 mg.
2) Increase total daily zinc intake to 30 mg.

Consult Part Two for information on substances, other than vitamins and minerals, said to accelerate wound healing, e.g., arginine, ornithine, aloe vera, DMSO, bioflavonoids, etc. Pay attention to the precautions.

Regimen for Those Exposed to High Levels of Environmental Pollutants

Overview

The pollutants in urban air, automobile exhausts and tobacco smoke all contain free radicals in abundance. Common air pollutants include nitrogen oxides and sulfur dioxide. When inhaled, these substances generate toxic oxygen forms that damage our tissues. Free-radical toxic oxygen forms have been implicated in accelerated aging, in cancer, heart disease and other maladies. People living in such urban areas as Los Angeles are often exposed to these noxious agents for prolonged periods. Antioxidant protection via supplements appears prudent.

The Regimen

Same as the Regimen for Smokers.

Regimen for Older People ("Senior Supplement")

Overview

The percentage of "senior citizens" (those sixty-five and over) is increasing rapidly in the United States. It is estimated that by the year 2000 there will be 31.8 million people in this age group in the U.S. alone. There are several reports indicating that many seniors consume inadequate diets and may have vitamin, mineral and protein-calorie deficiencies. Most of these studies have related to the aged poor and to those seniors who are living in institutions. But some studies show that even relatively affluent older people are at greater risk of nutritional deficiencies than the population as a whole.

In addition, older people are more likely than younger people to be taking various medications, some of which can predispose to nutritional deficiencies. Diuretics, for example, of the sort commonly used for the treatment of high blood pressure or congestive heart failure, can lead to deficiencies in potassium, magnesium, zinc and, conceivably, other nutrients. Potassium supplementation is given to diuretic users, but magnesium and zinc supplementation is still usually overlooked.

The elderly may have increased difficulty absorbing nutrients from their intestines—another factor that can adversely influence nutritional status with advancing years, again making supplementation more needed.

There are reports that the elderly may suffer from suboptimal zinc and chromium nutrition. Suboptimal zinc status could affect the immune system and be an important factor in the increased incidence of autoimmune diseases, cancer and infections that occur in the elderly. Suboptimal chromium status could be a factor in the decreased ability of the elderly to process glucose (decreased glucose tolerance).

The Basic Regimen for Men is recommended for senior men as an insurance supplement to protect against micronutrient deficiencies. (See Regimen for Postmenopausal Women for senior women.) Iron is not recommended, since iron deficiency in this group could reflect some underlying pathology that should be investigated and treated by a physician. (Supplementation with iron might "mask" the problem and delay treatment.) Seniors with hypercalcemia (high calcium in the blood) and those with renal failure (kidney failure) should not be taking calcium or magnesium supplementation, respectively. These latter patients are usually under medical supervision.

The Regimen

Women should follow the Regimen for Postmenopausal Women and men the Basic Regimen for Men except:

1) Total daily copper intake should be increased to 3 mg.
2) Total daily zinc intake should be increased to 30 mg.

Drug/Vitamin/Mineral Interactions

There are some combinations of drugs/vitamins/minerals that can be potentially dangerous or that can negate the effect of either the drugs or the nutrients. Read this section carefully, no matter which regimen you may be following.

ALCOHOL—Diminishes the stores or interferes with the body's absorption of thiamine, riboflavin, niacinamide, pyridoxine, folic acid, calcium, iron, zinc, magnesium, vitamins B_{12}, C, A and D. (See Regimen for Alcohol Drinkers.)

ANTACIDS—Over-the-counter aluminum-containing antacids may, if used regularly, interfere with the calcium status in bone. (See analysis of calcium, Part Two.)

ASPIRIN (and Other Anti-inflammatory Agents)—May interfere with the absorption and activity of vitamin C, folic acid and iron. Supplementation with any of the foregoing regimens should provide enough of these nutrients to overcome these adverse effects.

DILANTIN—This anticonvulsant may interfere with folic acid. Again, however, supplementation with any of the foregoing regimens should suffice to overcome this interference.

DIURETICS (Such as Hydrochlorothiazide and Furosemide)—May interfere with potassium, magnesium, zinc and result in deficiencies in all. Those who use any of the foregoing regimens should thereby obtain enough zinc and magnesium to overcome the adverse effects of these diuretics. Potassium should be taken only with a doctor's supervision.

ORAL CONTRACEPTIVES—May interfere, in particular, with pyridoxine (vitamin B_6) and folic acid. See Regimen for Women Using Oral Contraceptives, designed to eliminate potential drug-caused deficiencies.

STEROIDS—Chronic use of steroids can cause breakdown of protein in bone and produce osteoporosislike disorders. Supplemental calcium is needed, as provided in the foregoing regimens, to counteract these effects.

TETRACYCLINE—Chronic use may result in calcium deficiency. The antibiotic tetracycline, used regularly by some acne sufferers and others, binds with calcium and both get excreted from the body together. If you are using tetracycline regularly, take your calcium-containing supplement two or more hours before or after you take the tetracycline.

Some Special Cautionary Notes on Certain Drugs

—Users of *Isotretinoin* or *Accutane* for the treatment of cystic acne should avoid all vitamin A supplements while this drug is in use. Vitamin A supplements (including beta-carotene) may make your acne condition worse while using these drugs and/or increase adverse side effects from these drugs.

—Patients taking *levodopa* should restrict supplementary vitamin B_6 (pyridoxine) to less than 5 milligrams per day while taking this drug. B_6 converts levodopa into a form that cannot cross the blood/brain barrier, thus largely negating the desired effect of the drug, which is commonly used in Parkinsonism. Take the B_6 two hours before or after taking L-dopa. This will help prevent the drug from being converted into dopamine in the small intestine. (Dopamine is the form that cannot get through the blood/brain barrier.)

—Persons using the drug *Coumadin* should not consume supplementary vitamin K. Coumadin is an anticoagulant, and vitamin K antagonizes it.

For more information on drug/vitamin/mineral interactions, see: Ovensen, *Drugs*, 18:278, 1979; M. Winick, ed., *Nutrition and Drugs*, John Wiley and Sons, New York, 1983; D. A. Roe, *Drug-Induced Nutritional Deficiencies*, Avi Publishing Co., 1976; Drug-Nutrient Interaction Chart, Hoffmann-LaRoche, Inc.

twelve

FINDING THE RIGHT FORMULA ("One-a-Day," "Insurance," "Stress," etc.)

"Does It Matter Which Formula I Use?"

It's surprising how many people seem to believe that most vitamin/mineral products are the same or nearly the same—and that they all afford about equal protection. The fact is that there are literally hundreds of different formulations on the market and there are a great many differences among them in terms of quality, quantity of each ingredient, balance of composition, cost. A great many formulations appear to have been put together either without any scientific rationale whatsoever or with outdated, discredited information in mind. Many products come overloaded with certain vitamins—typically the B vitamins, providing doses that are much larger than necessary in some instances—while skimping or completely omitting other

312 THE COMPLETE GUIDE TO ANTI-AGING NUTRIENTS

needed nutrients. It is often obvious that quantities have been selected on an entirely arbitrary basis.

All of this says nothing about what is actually in the tablets— only what the manufacturer *claims* is in them. It isn't within the scope of this book to do chemical analyses of these products. I have carried out analyses of a sampling of products. There is some false labeling of content, but, in general, it appears that most products contain what they say they contain. (Claims made for those contents—that is, what the products can do for you—are, however, frequently misleading and often demonstrably untrue.) Future editions of this book may contain some actual analyses of product lines. For now, however, it is enough just to figure out how to get a product that offers the appropriate balance of nutrients.

There's such a confusing mélange of advertising claims that most people don't even know where to begin. I've seen many people who, in their desperation, throw up their hands and take nothing at all and others, in equal despair, who decide they had better "take one of everything." Much of the confusion has to do with whether one should take a "one-a-day," an "insurance" formula or a "stress" formula—or all three.

In the preceding chapter I've provided some guidelines for nutritional supplementation applicable to different life situations. Now, how do you go about getting supplements that will satisfy those guidelines? The answer is: You probably *won't* be able to satisfy them *exactly*. And it isn't necessary to do so. But I advise striving to come as close as possible. Let's look at some different ways of trying to do this.

The Single-Nutrient Approach

Every nutrient listed in the recommended regimens in the previous chapter can be purchased singly and in varying quantities. Thus one *could* put together one's own "super supplement" by buying each nutrient individually. That, however, would be an extremely costly, time-consuming and inconvenient way of approaching the problem. Furthermore, by taking all those individual tablets, capsules, etc., you would be exposing yourself to a lot of additional additives, dyes, preservatives and so on. In general, the single-nutrient approach is *not* recommended. You *can* use single-nutrient products to *supplement* your multivitamin/mineral or one-a-day preparation, to try to bring it up closer to what you're trying to achieve or in special situations recommended by your doctor. But if you have to add too many of these single nutrients to achieve your goal, you should give serious consideration to switching to an entirely different— more complete, better balanced—multivitamin/mineral product.

Again, use individual nutrient products only to help "bring up to snuff" multivitamin/mineral preparations that fall short of the goals outlined in the preceding chapter. And remember that it is usually better to fall a bit short of the goal than to exceed it in some particular. Balance is more important than quantity. The idea that if a small dose is good for you then a megadose must be even better has not been demonstrated.

The "One-a-Day" Approach

There are a great many "one-a-day" vitamin/mineral formulations that hundreds of thousands of Americans find convenient to use. Many physicians, in fact, get their own vitamin/mineral supplementation through these formulations, which require taking only *one* tablet or capsule daily.

The trouble is, it's difficult to get everything you really need into one pill. To put everything recommended in the Basic Regimens for Men and Women detailed in the preceding chapter, for example, would require a "horse pill," something so big you'd likely choke on it. One of the main reasons for this is that calcium and magnesium in the quantities needed/recommended are very bulky and would make one pill too large to take with anything approaching comfort.

One-a-days just can't deliver everything you need. And some are very poorly designed in terms of composition and balance of nutrients. Yet, by their very nature—given the claims implicit in the one-a-day philosophy—even the worst product will give the unwary consumer the impression he/she is doing everything that is necessary to protect nutritional health. The claim is: Just take your one-a-day and don't worry about nutritional deficiencies. If only it were that simple! It *isn't*.

I have another major objection to the one-a-days. I have

stressed throughout this book the need for antioxidant protection within the gastrointestinal tract where much oxidant damage can occur from the substances we ingest at each meal. It is far better to get your antioxidants in *divided* doses, preferably with *each* meal, rather than all at once in a one-a-day. In other words, the one-a-day approach is not very efficient. It puts a lot of nutrients into your system at one time; many of these may be wasted. Then, later in the day, when you need more protection, none is at hand. Dividing your supplement into three doses per day instead of taking it at once makes much more sense, enabling you to make far more efficient use of the nutrients while making protection more continuous.

Despite all these objections, I will not say categorically that you should not take a one-a-day product. I'm realistic enough to know that many individuals will not remember to take a supplement with each meal or will not want to go to that trouble. Some will say they don't want to take supplements three times a day because of expense. I will show you in the discussion of "insurance" formulas, however, that the cost of a truly adequate three-times-daily formula can actually be less than the cost of a generally inadequate one-a-day.

If the choice for you is between a one-a-day and nothing at all, then provided its composition is not too far out of balance, it's better to take the one-a-day. And if you've already stocked up on a year's supply of one-a-days, by comparing the formulation in your product with the proper regimen for you as described in the preceding chapter, you can supplement your one-a-days with single nutrients as discussed in the preceding section of this chapter.

Actually, a one-a-day *could* be designed that would require very little additional supplementation. My ideal one-a-day would and could contain (in one swallowable pill) all of the vitamins and minerals listed in the Basic Regimens in the indicated amounts—with the exception of calcium (magnesium would have to be limited to 200 milligrams). Supplementary calcium could then be taken from single-nutrient preparations.

There are dozens of one-a-day formulations on the market. I've examined a great many of these. They all fall far short of what I recommend in the preceding chapter, but, again, it is often better to take something than nothing at all, provided that something is not too badly designed. One of the best one-a-days I'm aware of is the Centrum High Potency Multivitamin/Mul--

timineral Formula from Lederle Laboratories, available without prescription. I cannot vouch for the product containing what it says it contains; I assume that Lederle is in fact delivering what it claims to be providing. The composition/balance of nutrients is much better here than in most of the one-a-days.

I am mentioning a few specific products to help guide you. Neither I nor any member of my family has any financial interest in or derives any financial interest, directly or indirectly, from any of the companies named. I recommend that you examine the composition of the products named and compare them with others. *It is entirely possible that you will find other products that come nearly as close or even closer to my recommendations as does Centrum.*

Each tablet of the Centrum formula contains:

Vitamin A (as acetate) in the amount of 5,000 IUs (100 percent of the U.S. RDA).

Vitamin E (as dl-alphatocopherol acetate) in the amount of 30 IUs (100 percent of the U.S. RDA).

Vitamin C (as ascorbic acid) in the amount of 90 milligrams (150 percent of the U.S. RDA).

Folic Acid in the amount of 400 micrograms (100 percent of the U.S. RDA).

Vitamin B_1 (as thiamine mononitrate) in the amount of 2.25 milligrams (150 percent of the U.S. RDA).

Vitamin B_2 (as riboflavin) in the amount of 2.6 milligrams (153 percent of the U.S. RDA).

Niacinimide in the amount of 20 milligrams (100 percent of the U.S. RDA).

Vitamin B_6 (as pyridoxine hydrochloride) in the amount of 3 milligrams (150 percent of the U.S. RDA).

Vitamin B_{12} (as cyanocobalamin) in the amount of 9 micrograms (150 percent of the U.S. RDA).

Vitamin D in the amount of 400 IUs (100 percent of the U.S. RDA).

Biotin in the amount of 45 micrograms (14 percent of the U.S. RDA).

Pantothenic Acid (as calcium pantothenate) in the amount of 10 milligrams (100 percent of the U.S. RDA).

Calcium (as dibasic calcium phosphate) in the amount of 162 milligrams (16 percent of the U.S. RDA).

Phosphorus (as dibasic calcium phosphate) in the amount of 125 milligrams (13 percent of the U.S. RDA).

Iodine (as potassium iodide) in the amount of 150 micrograms (100 percent of the U.S. RDA).

Iron (as ferrous fumarate) in the amount of 27 milligrams (150 percent of the U.S. RDA).

Magnesium (as magnesium oxide) in the amount of 100 milligrams (25 percent of the U.S. RDA).

Copper (as cupric oxide) in the amount of 3 milligrams (150 percent of the U.S. RDA).

Manganese (as manganese sulfate) in the amount of 7.5 milligrams (recommended in human nutrition but RDA not yet established).

Potassium (as potassium chloride) in the amount of 7.7 milligrams (RDA not established).

Chloride (as potassium chloride) in the amount of 7 milligrams (RDA not established).

Chromium (as chromium chloride) in the amount of 15 micrograms (RDA not established).

Molybdenum (as sodium molybdate) in the amount of 15 micrograms (RDA not established).

Selenium (from yeast) in the amount of 15 micrograms (RDA not established).

Zinc (as zinc sulfate) in the amount of 22.5 milligrams (150 percent of the U.S. RDA).

As I say, this is one of the best, i.e., most complete, one-a-days I've been able to find. Yet, you'll immediately spot shortcomings. If you will only consider taking a one-a-day, this one is pretty good. And it can be made better with individual nutrient supplementation. Zinc and copper are present in the proper ratio. Amounts of some of the nutrients, however, are so low that they appear to have been included just so they could show up on the label. This is typical of the one-a-day approach. Compare the contents listed above to the contents of the Basic Regimens outlined in the preceding chapter and you will immediately note the need for more vitamin A (and I recommend A in the form of beta-carotene), more E, more C, more calcium, more magnesium, more chromium and more selenium.

You may be tempted to think: Well, if my one-a-day isn't good enough by itself I'll just take it two or three times a day and not bother to switch to some other product. *Don't do that.* Taking a one-a-day such as the one above three times a day will still not provide the recommended doses of some of the nutrients, but you will end up taking *too much* of some other nutrients, throwing things even further out of balance. You could easily, for example, end up getting way too much vitamin D, folic acid, iron, manganese, etc. *Use your one-a-day once a day or don't use it at all.* If you want to supplement it, use single nutrients and do not exceed doses recommended in the previous chapter.

Better yet, give some thought to switching to an "insurance" formula.

The "Insurance" Approach

An "insurance" formula is one that contains at least the RDAs as well as the upper limits of safe and adequate doses of all the essential trace minerals, major minerals and vitamins. Insurance formulas, at their best, strive for a balance of nutrients that seems optimal given present knowledge. They are designed to help prevent the premature onset of degenerative diseases. The regimens detailed in the preceding chapter are all insurance formulas. They have the added benefit of being designed for use in divided doses; one or more tablets are taken with each meal, thus providing more continuous protection, especially antioxidant protection.

Unfortunately, though there are a great many one-a-day formulas, there are still very few products that qualify as insurance formulas. I believe we are just at the beginning of a trend that will result in a great many of these formulas within the next few years, but for now the choices are few. In fact, I have found only two insurance formulas that I can recommend. Again, however, you may be able to find others as good or even better.

One of these products is made by NutriGuard Research, a relatively new company started by an acquaintance of mine. I was consulted on a nonfee basis when this company researched its insurance formula. Again, however, neither I nor any member of my family has any financial interest, direct or indirect, in this company.

The product is called Broad Spectrum. Its one possible drawback—and it is more psychological than anything else—is that you take not one tablet a day but *nine*—three with each meal. The price, as of mid-1984, is $9.95 for 270 tablets, a month's supply. That is considerably less than the cost of a month's supply of many one-a-day products that provide far less protection.

Here is the formulation. A daily dose provides:

NUTRIENT	FORM	AMOUNT	% U.S. RDA
Vitamin A	beta-carotene	20,000 IU	400
Vitamin B_1	thiamine-HCL	10 mg	667
Vitamin B_2	riboflavin	10 mg	588
Niacinamide		100 mg	500
Pantothenic Acid	calcium pantothenate	50 mg	500
Vitamin B_6	pyridoxine-HCL	50 mg	2,500
Vitamin B_{12}	cyanoco-balamin	30 mcg	500
Folic Acid		400 mcg	100
Biotin		100 mcg	33
Vitamin C	ascorbic acid	1,000 mg	1,667
Vitamin D	ergocalciferol	400 IU	100
Vitamin E	d-alpha-toco-pherol acetate	400 IU	1,333
Vitamin K	phylloquinone	100 mcg	*
Choline	bitartrate	1,000 mg	*
Calcium	carbonate	1,000 mg	100
Magnesium	oxide	400 mg	100
Zinc	gluconate	30 mg	200
Iron	ferrous fumarate	18 mg	100
Manganese	gluconate	10 mg	*
Copper	gluconate	2 mg	100
Selenium	yeast	200 mcg	*
Chromium	yeast	100 mcg	*
Iodine	potassium iodide	150 mcg	100
Molybdenum	sodium molybdate	50 mg	*
Silicon	magnesium trisilicate	20 mg	*
Potassium	chloride	860 mg	*

* U.S. RDA not established.

Broad Spectrum is available in very few vitamin/mineral stores. In the interests of holding down costs to the consumer, NutriGuard sells the product by direct mail, both to physicians and to lay people. To obtain current order forms and other information, write:

NutriGuard Research
238 Lolita Street
Encinitas, California 92024

Another company that, in my view, makes some better-than-average products at lower-than-average costs is Bronson Pharmaceuticals. They sell two insurance formulas. One is called the Vitamin and Mineral Insurance Formula and the other is called the Fortified Vitamin and Mineral Insurance Formula. The fortified formula is considerably better than the basic formula. Bronson recommends six tablets daily, two with each meal. A bottle of 250 tablets, enough for six weeks, costs $15.30 as of mid-1984. Here's what six tablets daily provide:

NUTRIENT	FORM	AMOUNT	% U.S. RDA
Vitamin A	palmitate	15,000 IU	300
Vitamin D	cholecalciferol	400 IU	100
Vitamin E	dl-alphatoco-pherol acetate	400 IU	1,333
Vitamin K	phylloquinone	100 mcg	*
Vitamin C	ascorbic acid	2,500 mg	4,167
Vitamin B$_1$	thiamine mononitrate	20 mg	1,333
Vitamin B$_2$	riboflavin	20 mg	1,176
Vitamin B$_6$	pyridoxine-HCL	30 mg	1,500
Vitamin B$_{12}$	cobalamin	90 mcg	1,500
Niacinamide		200 mg	1,000
Pantothenic Acid	D-calcium pantothenate	150 mg	1,500
Biotin		3,000 mcg	1,000
Folic Acid		400 mcg	100
Choline	bitartrate	500 mg	*
Calcium	phosphate	250 mg	25

NUTRIENT	FORM	AMOUNT	% U.S. RDA
Phosphorus	phosphate	250 mg	25
Magnesium	oxide	200 mg	50
Iron	fumarate	30 mg	167
Zinc	gluconate	30 mg	200
Copper	gluconate	2 mg	100
Iodine	kelp	150 mcg	100
Manganese	gluconate	10 mg	*
Molybdenum	sodium molybdate	200 mcg	*
Chromium	yeast	200 mcg	*
Selenium	yeast	100 mcg	*
Inositol		500 mg	*
Rutin		200 mg	*
Para-amino-benzoic Acid		30 mg	*

* U.S. RDA not established.

This is a good insurance formula, although I would prefer that vitamin A be provided in the form of beta-carotene, which has extremely low toxicity. Some nutrients are provided in amounts above that which I believe is necessary, while calcium and magnesium are provided in amounts lower than those I believe to be optimal.

For more information and current order forms, write:

Bronson Pharmaceuticals
4526 Rinetti Lane
La Canada, California 91011

Bronson, incidentally, is a good source for vitamin C in crystal (powder) form, which is the purest, least expensive way of obtaining it.

"Stress" Formulas

The so-called "stress" formulas have become very popular lately thanks to heavy advertising. These formulas contain the B vitamins, vitamin C and occasional minerals, such as zinc, and some of the other vitamins. The emphasis, however, is on the

B vitamins, which are often included in megadoses (greater than ten times the RDAs). Emphasis is often also placed on vitamin C. These formulas are supposed to help you cope with the stresses of daily life and with such traumas as infection and surgery. They are often pitched at the chronic "workaholic."

The truth is, there is no truly scientific rationale for the stress formulas. They are the product of hype rather than of any real need. You are far better off taking an insurance formula than one of these poorly designed, typically unbalanced "stress" products.

Other Formulas

There are now formulas for almost every situation you can imagine. One recent brochure I received has an "anti-arthritic formula," an "antihypertensive formula," a "cardiovascular formula," an "immune-system (antiviral) formula," a "sleep formula," a "dieter's formula," an "antidepressant formula" and an "antifatigue formula." *Be extremely wary of any formula that claims to counteract any particular disease.* Claims made for most of these formulas cannot be substantiated. Moreover, most of the special formulas I've surveyed are very poorly designed. A basic regimen of the sort recommended in the previous chapter, with variations for different situations, will provide better results. The name of the game in the supplement supermarket these days is to keep on inventing new "needs" for vitamins/minerals. If you believed all the claims, you'd be taking at least a couple dozen separate formulas, jeopardizing your health in the process. Vitamin and mineral supplementation *can* help prevent some diseases but not with the specificity that these different formulas imply. By trying these different formulas you not only waste your money but you also get off the track of a good, basic micronutritional program. Most of the specialized formulas I've seen are more likely to *create* problems than to relieve them.

thirteen

CONSUMER CONCERNS: QUESTIONS AND ANSWERS

Q—What are the most important things to look for on a product label?

A—First you'll want to look to see what's in the product. If you're looking for an acceptable one-a-day or a good insurance formula, you'll want to note quantities and the balance of nutrients. Compare these with the regimens I recommended at the beginning of this section. You'll also want to pay attention to the source of each nutrient, which is usually shown in parentheses right after the name of the nutrient. Again, compare with the information provided earlier. Pay attention to what _isn't_ in the product, too. Are there some things that should be there that are entirely missing? Check out the list of additives. Use common sense here; if you can find a similar product with far fewer additives, buy that one. And when it comes to comparing cost, don't just look at price. You must look at price in terms of number of tablets or capsules in the container _and_ in terms of the amount of nutrient in each tablet or capsule. Bottles of the same product put out by different manufacturers may be about the same size and still contain significantly different amounts of nutrients. If there are very large differences in price, check the labels again. One may be much more expensive because it is chelated or in timed-release form. (See information on these below.) Check seals to make sure that the product is tightly capped for freshness. Do not be swayed by "brand name." Just because you've seen a product heavily advertised does not mean that it is any better than a less-advertised product. Look for an expiration date and don't buy beyond that date. The lack of an expiration date, however, should not be any cause for rejecting the product. Most products sell well before their potency is compromised by having been on the shelf too long. Be wary of products that make excessive claims related to specific diseases or that promise weight loss, increased sexual potency, enhanced energy, etc. Such claims have not been substantiated and should make the product suspect from a scientific point of view.

Q—How can I be sure the vitamins, minerals and other supplements I buy are fresh and have full potency?

A—Unfortunately, you cannot be absolutely certain of this. If you look carefully at the labels on some products you will find an "expiration date" beyond which you should not buy the product. There are a few companies that stress the "freshness" and "potency" of their products and "guarantee" same through certain dates. Whether these guarantees really have any practical value is doubtful. Most products will, in fact, sell well before their potency is seriously compromised. The products that boast of full potency and freshness in expensive full-color ads tend, not surprisingly, to be higher priced than a lot of other products, and there is no evidence they really are any fresher. Look for expiration dates on labels but don't be alarmed if you don't find any. (Inclusion of expiration dates is not required.) Instead, look for a good outer and inner seal on product bottles and be cautious about buying from the bargain bin; products therein may very likely have been on the shelf too long.

Q—Once I've opened a bottle of vitamins or minerals should I store the container in the refrigerator?

A—No. Keep supplements in a dry, dark place away from sunlight and heat, but don't put them in the refrigerator, where dampness may damage them. Keep lids tightened when not in use; buy products that are packaged in opaque containers that will not permit easy penetration by sunlight. If you buy a large container, you might consider putting a supply good for a couple of weeks or a month in a smaller opaque container so that you are not constantly exposing your main supply to fresh air each time you open the bottle or jar. Some supplements, for example, oil-based ones, will age more quickly than others. It's best to buy these supplements in smaller quantities so that you use them up before they rancidify. And if you buy large quantities of vitamin C, yeasts or other supplements in powder, granular, or loose form, be sure to follow the instructions above regarding use of large quantities of supplements.

Q—Are "natural" vitamins really better than "synthetic" ones? And if the label doesn't say "natural" should I assume the product is synthetic?

A—This is one of the most confusing issues facing the consumer. And many supplement manufacturers have done everything they can to take advantage of that confusion. Consumers all over the world are being persuaded to pay far more for natural food-supplement products than for synthetic ones. The advertising claims imply that only the natural products provide full potency and that the synthetic products are somehow "bad" or deficient. Many of the natural vitamin C products, for example, actually contain only a small amount of ascorbic acid derived from natural sources. A "rose hip" vitamin C is generally 90 percent or more synthetic. Moreover, the so-called natural products go through most of the same "unnatural" processing procedures that the synthetic ones do. *The fact is, in any event, that natural and synthetic versions of the same substance are necessarily chemically identical.* There is absolutely no reason, therefore, to expect that the action of the two versions will be different in any respect. When pressed to the wall, many of the advocates of natural supplements are forced to concede this point, but then they sometimes try to fall back on the argument that other substances—"natural contaminants"—are necessary for the supplement to do its job properly and that these natural substances are removed in the process of making synthetic supplements. If there were any truth to this convenient argument at least a few of those "contaminants" would long since have been identified and recognized to be as important as the vitamins and minerals themselves. It is often claimed, for instance, that the bioflavonoids are necessary for vitamin C to work optimally. There is no support for this idea. On the contrary, a study cited earlier in this book showed just the opposite to be true—that synthetic vitamin C utterly devoid of bioflavonoids was absorbed more readily by the human body than natural vitamin C in combination with bioflavonoids. In addition to all this, there are some risks involved in consuming large quantities of supplements derived from natural sources. *Some* bone meal and desiccated liver products, used as sources of natural B vitamins and various minerals, for example, have been shown to contain potentially hazardous levels of various contaminants, including pesticides, heavy metals, etc. *Don't pay extra for "natural" supplements and, in fact, be suspicious of those products that make great claims for their "natural" origins.*

Q—What about products that claim to be "organic" in origin or derived from "organically grown" materials?

A—Well, if you're buying fruits or vegetables or grain products that are said to be organically grown, this *may* mean that they were not exposed to a lot of pesticides or other chemicals. But, in fact, "organic" in this context has no real scientific or legal definition; it may mean whatever a manufacturer or retailer chooses to make it mean. So before you buy anything labeled "organic," at least ask the seller exactly what is implied. Most of what I've stated above with respect to "natural" applies here. The only real definition for organic is the one used in science; any compound that contains carbon is organic. Thus even most plastics are organic. Don't be taken in by this terminology. I'd think twice before I'd buy any product labeled "organic" vitamins or minerals. The fact that a manufacturer utilizes this kind of ill-defined labeling might make me lose confidence in that company's scientific integrity.

Q—Are products that claim to be free of artificial preservatives, dyes, etc. better than others?

A—It depends upon what others you are comparing them to; if everything else is equal I would certainly prefer a product that was not loaded down with preservatives and artificial colors. Examine labels carefully and avoid those products that seem to have a long list of additives, such as coloring agents; preservatives, binders, fillers. There is some speculation that additives may cause serious health problems in people who take megadose quantities of supplements containing these extraneous substances. They may not cause problems in small amounts, but when you ingest enough of them, a variety of adverse reactions, including a number of allergies, may arise.

Q—Is it really necessary to worry about quality control in supplements? Doesn't the FDA monitor all that for us?

A—The Food and Drug Administration requires that supplement manufacturers list all of the ingredients that go into their products. Manufacturers who fail to do this or who do not deliver what they say they are delivering on their labels can get into legal difficulty if detected. In fact, however, monitoring is sporadic and compliance uneven. It is my impression, based on some chemical analyses, that most manufacturers deliver what they say they do, in terms of nutrient content. Advertising claims, however, are frequently unsubstantiated and often outrageous. The FDA seems to be fighting an uphill battle trying to keep up with the flood of supplements coming into the market. So the answer is: No, you can't count on the FDA to completely ensure product integrity or safety. Vitamins, minerals and other nutritional supplements definitely do not receive the scrutiny or testing that pharmaceuticals do. And the fact that an advertising claim goes unchallenged by the FDA should not lead you to believe that the claim has been substantiated.

Q—I've heard that mineral supplements do no good unless they are chelated. Is this true and what does it mean?

A—A number of supplement products are advertised as "chelated." These products usually cost more than nonchelated products. Chelation is a process that is supposed to make minerals more readily absorbable by altering their electrical charge. There is little evidence that chelated minerals are worth their extra price. The bioavailability of nonchelated minerals is sufficient when taken in the sort of combinations/regimens recommended earlier in this book. No need to spend extra money on chelated products.

Q—What is the best form in which to take supplements— pills, capsules, powders?

A—This may depend upon the individual supplement and the individual consumer. There are some people, for example, who cannot swallow pills without choking or panicking. Obviously those people need another way of taking supplements. Pills and tablets are best for most people. Nutrients can be tightly bound together in this form and protected against oxidation and rancidification. Fat-soluble vitamins such as vitamins A, E and D, on the other hand, are often conveniently packaged in gelatin capsules, and these are fine too. The capsules, in fact, often obviate the need for additional preservatives because they provide such a good seal by themselves. Powders, crystals, granules are often the forms in which vitamin C is sold in larger quantities. Generally these forms will have no additives at all, which is certainly an advantage. Cost is usually lower, too. Some manufacturers are now producing "insurance" formulas made up of all the needed vitamins and minerals in powder form that can be mixed with juices and the like. And drops are also available for those who can't tolerate pills or capsules.

Q—Are "timed-release" capsules or tablets worth spending extra money on?

A—It's difficult to know how well most of these work. Do they in fact dissolve at the rates claimed? I don't think they are worth their higher price. The idea of getting continuous antioxidant protection is an important one, but you can achieve satisfactory results by taking your insurance formula in divided doses, ideally three times a day, once with each meal (see recommendations earlier in this book). That will provide you with ongoing protection without the need for more expensive and not entirely predictable timed-release formulations. Another major drawback to the timed-release products is that they come in a very limited number of formulations. You want to pick your supplements first for their overall design—content and balance—and not for convenience of ongoing "release."

Q—There seem to be all kinds of different forms of various vitamins; how do I know which is best?

A—I have listed the cheapest and most bioavailable forms of the various nutrients I recommend at the beginning of this section. I strongly recommend, for example, that vitamin A be taken in the form of beta-carotene and not as preformed vitamin A (in the form of fish oil, for example), which can be quite toxic in high doses in some individuals who use it for prolonged periods. I have provided the form I believe is best for each vitamin and mineral. Special confusion prevails with respect to vitamin

C. Labels may indicate that vitamin C is "derived from" everything from palm to corn to rose hips. What you want to be aware of is *how much* of the vitamin you are getting. This is more important than where it is coming from. I've already discussed the "natural" versus "synthetic" issue, which, again, plagues vitamin C in particular. The best way to get your vitamin C is in a good "insurance" formula. And if you want to add more to your daily regimen, the best form is a pure crystal or granular form—best because it's cheapest and purest. A source from which you can buy vitamin C in this form has been provided in the preceding chapter. Vitamin E is another nutrient that comes in many different forms. Stick to those products that get vitamin E from alpha-tocopherol. "Mixed tocopherols," another source of vitamin E, include forms for which there is no evidence of nutritional benefit. For further information, see the recommended regimens at the beginning of this section as well as the individual analyses of each nutrient in Part Two.

Q—Are hair-analysis tests a good way of determining which supplements a person needs?

A—Claims are made that analysis of hair will yield information on mineral stores in the body. Unfortunately, hair analysis is a highly unreliable means of determining any mineral deficiency. Apart from the fact that mineral content of hair does not necessarily reflect mineral content in bodily tissue, there are all sorts of variables that can bias the results of these tests. In general, unless there is reason to suspect a particular vitamin/mineral deficiency, you can best determine your micronutrient needs by reading the analyses of the various nutrients in Part Two and by reviewing the recommended "insurance" regimens. If you suspect a genuine nutritional deficiency after reading the symptoms in Part Two, there are a variety of medical tests that can be performed or ordered by your doctor.

INDEX

acatalasemia, 152
Accutane, 310
acetylcholine, 221–22, 281
acidophilus, 77, 263
acne:
   vitamin A and, 310
   vitamin B_6 and, 99
   zinc and, 193
actinic keratosis, 248
adenine, 214–15
adenosine, 74, 218
adenosine triphosphate (ATP), 160, 303
adrenal-gland hormone production, 104
adriamycin, reducing toxicity of, 182
Agent Orange poisoning, 91, 93
aging:
   delaying morbidity in, 15, 21–22, 24
   economic impact of, 20
   life-span and, 14–15, 20–21, 34
   "magic bullets" for, 14–15
   as product of accumulated abuses, 22–23
   schoolchildren's perceptions on, 19–20
   theories of, 28–33
   variability of, 22
   see also life-span
AIDS (acquired immune deficiency syndrome), 99, 189, 202
alcohol consumption, 23, 25, 41, 48, 55, 304–5, 309
   calcium and, 70, 304
   cancer and, 48, 52

magnesium deficiency and, 160, 304, 309
   moderation in, 48
   supplementation regimen for, 304–305, 309
   vitamin A and, 304
   vitamin B_1 (thiamine) and, 304, 305
   vitamin B_2 and, 304, 305
   vitamin B_6 and, 99, 304
   vitamin C and, 117, 304, 305
   vitamin E and, 304, 305
   zinc and, 304, 305
   see also folic acid
aldehydes, 206
alfalfa sprouts, 54
allicin, 248
aloe vera, 77, 263–64
alpha-one-antitrypsin, 143
Alzheimer's disease, 74, 221–23, 288–289
Ames Test, 260
amines, 174, 236
amino acids, 73–74, 198–213
ammonium molybdate, 172
anemia:
   from copper deficiency, 142
   in elderly, 157
   in infants, 155
   from iron deficiency, 150–52, 154, 155, 159
   molybdenum and, 175
   pernicious, 21, 103, 151–52
   testing for, 159
   from vitamin B_6 deficiency, 96
   vitamin B_{12} and, 103, 152